Hair Loss Solutions

Causes, Prevention and Treatments

Jonathan Affleck

Hair Loss Solutions

Causes, Prevention and Treatments

ISBN-13: 978-1512390247

ISBN-10: 1512390240

Disclaimer

This book is for information purposes only. While every attempt has been made to verify the information provided in this book, neither the author nor the publisher assumes any responsibility for errors or omissions.

The information, ideas, and suggestions in this book are not intended as a substitute for professional medical advice. Before following any suggestions contained in this book, you should consult your personal physician. Neither the author nor the publisher shall be liable or responsible for any loss or damage allegedly arising as a consequence of your use or application of any information or suggestions in this book.

Table of Contents

1. Introduction

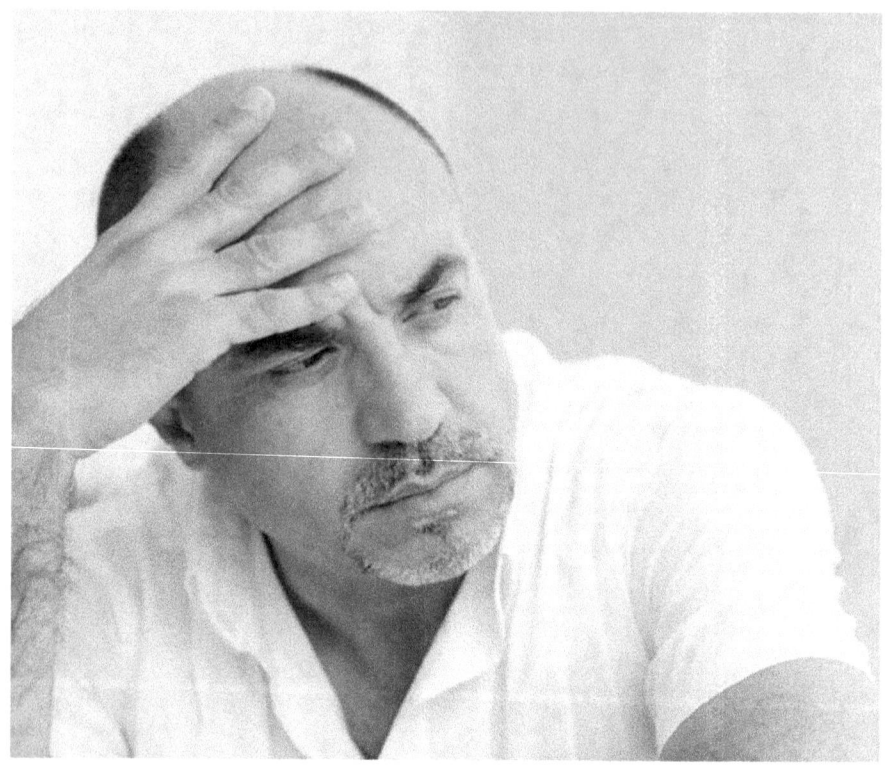

Hundreds of millions of people all over the world are suffering from hair loss and some of them are in a desperate search for a cure. Loss of hair makes you feel much older than your actual age and for some, hair loss leads to loss of self-esteem and confidence. Unfortunately, there are so many causes of hair loss today but the good news is that there are also so many treatment options as well and you don't have to deal with this problem for ever. The best thing to do when experiencing hair loss is to book an appointment with a doctor and have your condition checked. Hair loss can be a side effect of medications or it could even be the result of a more serious medical condition. Other causes include lifestyle, genetic problem and use of wrong products and so on.

Successful treatment of hair loss is only possible if you know the actual cause of the problem. By understanding your unique situation, you will thus be able to identify the best hair treatment options for your condition. Even though there is nothing much you can do about genetics, there are so many treatments that can help keep your hair shiny and healthy. Some medications will work pretty well for common hair causes. For cases that are more severe, you will need to consider other options of concealing the loss such as using a wig. If you are thinking of a permanent solution, you might as well consider going for a hair transplant. There are also over the counter medications and natural treatments that can prove useful to your condition as well. As such, the most important thing is to understand about your unique situation and explore the treatment options that work best for you.

Having your hair turn out exactly the way you desire is definitely an achievable possibility. This book will show you how you can do this by providing you with unique information ranging from hair loss causes to treatment options available and helpful tips and advice to help you contain the situation. However, remedying hair loss issues is not an overnight affair but calls for a lot of patience and dedication. While some will manage to restore their hair within some few weeks, it might takes months and years for others to achieve the same results.

2. Hair Loss: A Primer

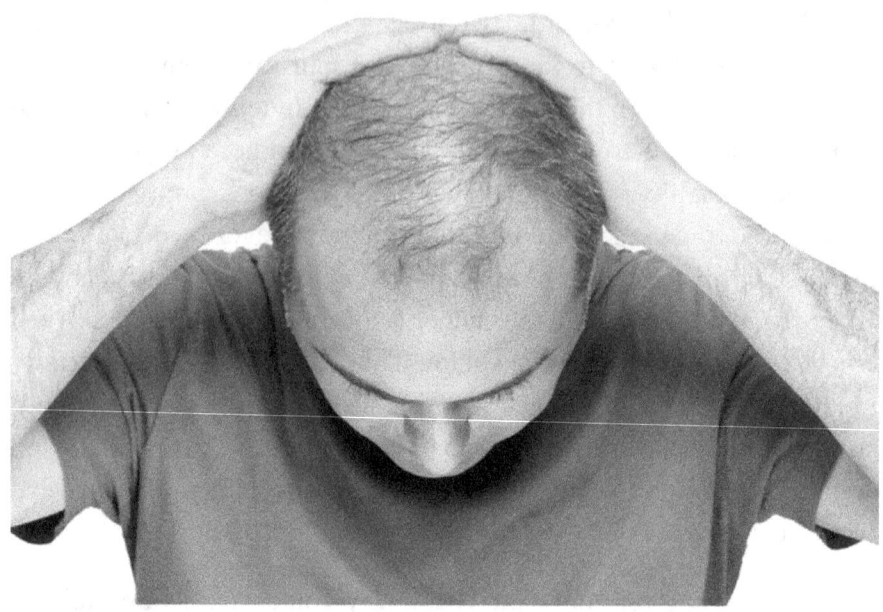

Hair is by far much more complex than it simply appears on the skin surface. Besides playing a key role on how men and women appear, hair also helps in transmission of sensory information and is responsible for gender identification. When a fetus is 22 weeks old, all its hair follicles are already formed on its body. During this development stage, the fetus has nearly 5 million hair follicles all over its body. The head has about 1 million with the scalp alone having about 100000 hair follicles. Since new hair follicles are not generated within the course of human lives, the 5 million hair follicles is the maximum number.

The average human scalp has 100,000 hair follicles. After birth, there is no formation of new follicles. Both men and women lose an average of between 50 and 100 hairs in a day. A loss of at least 150 hairs per day consistently is considered to be a significant loss of hair. However, what really leads to hair loss remains a mystery and hair specialists do not even agree on the actual causes of hair loss.

Hair loss is described as alopecia which implies hair loss from the body or head. At a certain point in their lives, both men and women suffer from thinning and loss of hair, a condition triggered by many factors ranging from hormones, age and genetics.

Miniaturization or hair thinning is the first hair loss stage. Growth of hair largely depends on whether or not the hair follicle is functioning properly. In a normal circumstance, hair growth takes place in a cycle which include anagen and telogen phase which are the growth and resting phases respectively.

Hair thinning comes with aging and it results from the complex interaction of hormones and genes. Also, as people age, hair growth rate tends to slow down as well. Hair loss or alopecia generally comes in different forms as detailed here below.

Involutional alopecia refers to the natural condition where the hair thins gradually with age. As more hair follicles enter into a resting phase, remaining hairs tend to become fewer in number and shorter in length. Androgenic alopecia is generally a genetic condition which affects men and women alike.

In men, the condition is known as the male pattern baldness and can start during teenage or early 20's and leads to a considerable loss of hair. It is characterized by receding hairline as well as disappearance of hair gradually from the frontal scalp and crown. This condition is also present in women and is referred to as female pattern baldness but occurs in their late 40s.

Alopecia areata is a form of hair loss that starts suddenly causing patchy hair loss among children and in young adults. The condition can easily result in baldness but there is also a high likelihood that hair will return within some few years. Then there is alopecia universal, a condition where hair from all over the body falls out. This includes eyelashes, public hair and eyebrows.

Most children also experience trichotillomania which is a kind of psychological disorder whereby a person tends to pull his or her own hair. Hair can also thin out temporarily over the scalp through a condition known as the telogen effluvium. This is normally caused by changes in hair growth cycles. At the same time, lots of hair also enters in a resting phase which causes subsequent hair thinning and shedding.

Even though hair loss is generally surrounded by many mysteries, the medical and scientific community has developed numerous approaches that help in dealing with hair loss and promoting restoration of lost hair.

3. Major Causes of Hair Loss

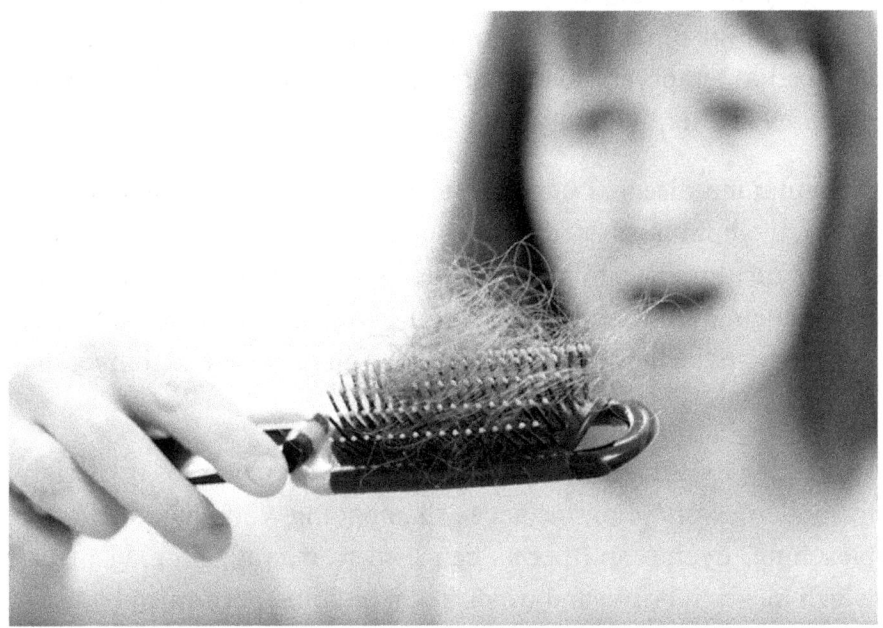

Doctors and researchers alike are yet to find out why some hair follicles have a relatively shorter growth period compared to others. Hair loss is caused by a range of several factors. For starters, hormones are largely responsible for hair loss among most people, especially when androgen hormone is present in abnormal levels in the human body. This male hormone is produced by both women and men and plays a critical role in hair loss.

Hair loss is also influenced greatly by genes from both parents. Genes influence the predisposition of a person to either female or male pattern baldness. Temporary hair loss can also result from stress and illness. Emotional disorders and stress not only causes weight loss but also hair loss as well. Fungal infection also causes ringworms in the body which leads to loss of hair.

Drugs especially chemotherapy drugs which are used to treat cancer highly contribute to hair loss. This is also caused by birth control pills and blood thinners as well as beta adrenergic blockers which are used in treatment of blood pressure. X- Rays, injuries and burns can lead to temporary loss of hair. In this case, normal hair growth is achieved after the injury has healed.

Autoimmune diseases can lead to alopecia areata. This condition makes the immune system to rev up for reasons that are not known. This greatly affects hair follicles. However, most people experiencing alopecia areata tend to have their hair growing back even though the new hair might have a lighter color and thinner than normal hair.

Cosmetic procedures have been a major cause of hair loss especially in modern work. For instance, shampooing your hair too often, bleaching, dyeing and perms can lead to overall thinning of hair which makes it brittle and weak. Tight braiding performed by use of hot curlers or rollers can break and damage the hair. However, most of these procedures are not likely to result in complete baldness. In case the problem is removed, the hair is likely to grow back again normally. But if the scalp or hair is severely damaged, this can lead to permanent bald patches.

Medical conditions are also major causes of hair loss like thyroid disease, diabetes, lupus, and anemia and iron deficiency. However, after the underlying medical condition has been treated, hair will return. Doctors say that there is a particular disease known as alopecia areata which attacks hair follicles and causes hair loss. Thyroid disease is yet another medical condition that can lead to loss of hair. Thyroid glands play a major role of regulating hormones and fluctuating hormone problems can lead to hair loss. A poor diet/ nutrition will cause hair loss as well especially low protein diets.

Medications used to treat diseases also have undesirable side effects with hair loss being one of them. Some medications are known to cause changes in hair color, texture and sometimes even loss of hair. The extent of hair loss caused by medication will depend on the specific drugs being taken and their side effects.

3.1 Genetics

Genetic hair loss, otherwise referred to as androgenetic alopecia is a condition that has been surrounded by many theories and misconceptions. In fact, there is a popular myth among people that hair loss problems are passed on to men from their mother's family side while women get hair loss problems from the father's family side. There are so many other myths that try to explain how hair loss is passed on from one generation to the other.

While scientists agree that the common male pattern baldness is based on genetics and that it is not possible to suffer from common baldness without specific inherited genes being present, the truth is that the genes are passed on to children from either of the two parent. However, the specific kind of inheritance as well as the role played by each parent still remains unclear. While most of the theoretical models propose on focusing on a specific dominant gene, one thing that is still clear is that genetic hair loss is ideally a polygenic trait. This means it is a very complex condition that most likely involves a myriad of genes.

Even in the midst of these ambiguities surrounding genetic hair loss, it is an undeniable fact that DHT or dihydrotestosterone has a major role to play in this. DHT is a male sex hormone/ androgen produced by men and women. With men producing mores testosterone than women, this has largely been suspected to be the main difference on how women and men respond to effects of DHT on the hair follicles and the rest of the body. Women experience hair loss all over their scalp as their hairline from remains largely unaffected. For men, hair loss happens at the hairline front and temples including the top of head as well.

As such, men are easily diagnosed with the androgenetic alopecia condition than women who normally experience hair loss as a result of hormonal changes during pregnancy and stress. As far as the genetic causes of androgenetic alopecia are concerned, it is not entirely clear what hormone level can trigger hair loss or what can make the hair loss worse. Gene expression related to genetic hair loss is affected by a wide range of factors such as hormone levels, stress and age. Also, just because you have baldness genes, this doesn't mean the condition must manifest itself.

Understanding genetic hair loss has key implications when it comes to diagnosing and treating baldness. Early diagnosis for instance can be used to minimize the risk of suffering from baldness. However, the good thing is that genetic hair loss is preventable and treatable if the right products are used. In fact, you don't have to go through rigorous treatments like hair transplant to treat genetic hair loss provided it is diagnosed early enough.

3.2 Age

As we age, the functions of the body deteriorates gradually. Genetics also have a critical role in influencing the response of the body to aging. Aging occurs differently among people and while some lose hearing and sight as they grow, others manifest signs of baldness and hair loss. As such, researchers have concluded that there seems to be a strong association between age and hair loss.

Testosterone has been largely blamed to be the major cause of male pattern baldness. Cells are affected by presence of testosterone hormone in the body as they start to age. Hair follicles start to manifest signs of declined activity. With the cellular activity continuing to reduce with age, the hair starts thinning and falling out. However, this situation is not present among young people as they lack testosterone hormone even though this doesn't result to balding. In fact, medical professionals and researchers have never understood the actual mechanism involved in balding. It is simply known that hair loss is caused by hormones why baldness begins at an older age has never been understood exactly.

As the body continues to age, the blood circulatory system gets less efficient and oxygen is not well delivered to the body extremities. This reduces the amount of oxygen that certain limbs and the scalp receives. With reduced oxygen delivery to the scalp, hair follicles receive a little amount of oxygen. As a result, the hair follicles have low energy and end up dying as a result. With reduced energy in the hair follicles, they are unable to divide normally and their growth is hampered as well. In the long run, the amount of hair being produced reduces which ends up causing hair loss.

Also, the body has a natural tendency of directing most of its energy towards areas that need the energy most. With age, people tend to do little physical activities which cause most of the tissues in the body to regress since their use is highly minimized. This is exactly what befalls the hair. As we age, amount of oxygen the body delivers to the hair reduces as the scalp doesn't need as much energy as such. The body focuses more on supplying oxygen to other areas of the body that need it most and this leads to hair thinning and falling.

Even though it is not deniable that there is a certain association between hair loss and age, this link can be broken. It is possible to maintain a good growing hair even at your advanced stages in life. It all depends on your lifestyle and how good you take care of your hair. There also certain drugs like Finasteride that are used to boost the functions of hair follicles so that they can still continue with hair production even in an advanced age. Additionally, you can also improve hair growth using alternative remedies like herbs and minimize hair loss at old age. These medications boost circulatory of blood to hair follicles and eliminate toxins that hinder hair growth.

3.3 Hormone Effect

It is widely known that there is a connection between hormone and hair loss. Normally, as we age, the hormones in our bodies also change as well. This affects the body in a big way as a whole and hair loss is one of the consequences of hormonal changes. But what exactly happens with hormones? At the most basic aspect of it, hormonal changes increase the speed of hair loss. Changes and loss of hormones ends up confusing the body even more which makes it to respond in different ways.

The good thing is that you can address hormonal changes in your body and tame the extent of hair loss in the process. The problems associated with changes in hormones are those that happen in daily life and can thus be handled easily. Hormonal related hair loss is known to be more significant in women than in men. Naturally, women are known to be hormonal creatures and fluctuation of hormones in their body is normal. While this is partly attributed to their monthly cycle, hormonal change is a natural process that happens in all life stages.

For instance, most women experience accelerated hair loss at the end of a pregnancy and the next six months. This is a period when the body is resetting its levels of hormone and as this happens, the hair will gradually fall out. After delivery, the body suddenly resets itself, hair stops growing and it is shed off. However, this is quite normal. Women also experience an increased hair fall during menopause. This has been attributed to the reduced production of estrogen which the body has been depending on but can no longer produce it.

As you can see, hair loss related to hormones is quite natural, at least to some extent. Nevertheless, most people are quite uncomfortable with it especially when it starts to get extreme. If the problem continues for a period of 6 months, this indicates that there is a deeper problem with your hormones and the hair loss might be a sign of a more serious problem. Complicated and deep hormone issues are major causes of hair loss but are not easily identifiable. Sometimes, acne occurs alongside hair loss and most of the hair falls due to DHT, a highly concentrated male hormone which healthy women shouldn't have.

It is also interesting to note that your behavior or mood can lead to hormonal malfunction. The good thing is that you can deal with hormonal changes and thus contain your hair loss. There is a wide range of medicines and vitamin supplements that you can use to control your hormones while reducing hair loss as well. As such, ensure that you take a daily dosage of multi vitamin as well as omega 3 fish oil so that your hair can remain intact. The earlier you deal with your hormonal changes the better as this will help prevent a lot of hair from being lost and help avoid other problems associated with hormonal malfunction.

3.4 Common Diseases That Cause Hair Loss

In the medical world, hair loss is known as alopecia. Hair loss can at times be the effect of another disease or illness. Further down, alopecia is classified to scarring and the non scarring conditions. Scarring alopecia involves the permanent growth of hair follicles with no chances of re- growth. One of the common diseases that cause hair loss is alopecia areata. This autoimmune disease causes circular hair loss spots and mostly runs in families. It results from the hair follicles being attached by white blood cells. Loss of hair in this regard can involve presence of patches on beard and head as well as complete hair loss on the scalp. However, more often than not, hair can re-grow back without any treatment.

Another condition that leads to widespread hair shedding is telogen effluvium. This happens after many hair follicles enter the rest cycle prematurely. Often, the condition is caused by traumatic events such as acute illness, major surgery, hormonal changes, big life changes and anesthesia. However, this is not a permanent condition and hair tends to grow again. Another disease is tinea capitis, a fungal infection largely responsible for hair loss among children. Its major symptoms include presence of white scaly flakes or large blisters covering the scalp. Also, some children experience swelling of lymph nodes under their years.

Thyroid disease is yet another very common cause of hair loss. Thyroid gland is responsible for regulation of metabolism in the body. If your thyroid gland is under or over active, this can affect growth of hair which becomes sparse and thin or brittle, sparse and dry. However, after the thyroid problem has been treated, growth of hair should return to normality. Dietary problems also cause hair loss to a greater extent especially due to diseases like anemia, malnutrition, diabetes, bulimia and anorexia.

Various medications used in treating most of these diseases also cause alopecia. The most common medications causing hair loss are drugs used to treat cancer. For instance, chemotherapy accelerates hair loss even though its effects might not be long lasting. After the treatment has been complete, growth of hair will begin. Another autoimmune disease called lupus leads to inflammation of organ tissues in the body. 50 percent of people suffering from lupus experience hair loss which can be either temporary or permanent and is characterized by a patchy head.

Scarring alopecia leads to an invisible scarring below the scalp with the hair follicles being replaced with a scar tissue. The condition is caused by the attack of hair follicles and the skin by the immune system and can result in permanent loss of hair. There are several other diseases that can cause hair loss. Depending on the disease, this can be a permanent or temporary condition. Different diseases affect growth of hair in various ways and while some cause small baldness spots on the head, others result in total hair loss. Since alopecia is treatable, it is advisable that you seek medical assistance to deal with the problem.

4. How to Cope with Hair Thinning

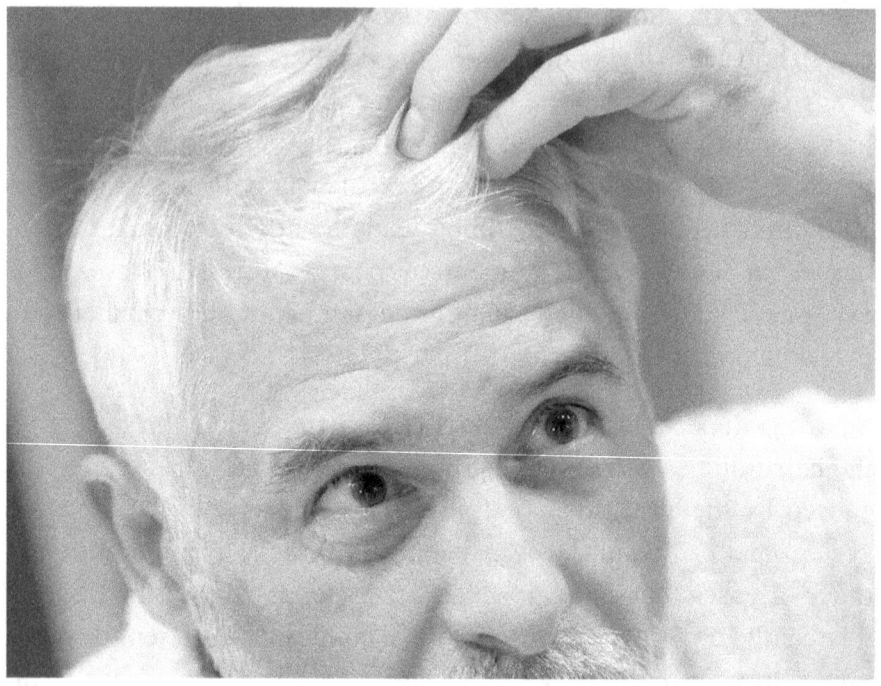

One of the most difficult things to handle in life is hair thinning especially due to the fact that it alters one's appearance. In fact, many men and women have ended up losing their self confidence and esteem when the crowning glory is gone. The most important thing in coping with hair thinning is to know the reasons behind it. According to hair specialists and professionals, hair thinning can either be a temporary or permanent condition. Pattern hair thinning or permanent thinning of hair is present among people whose parents have exactly the same problem. In most cases, the problem is usually a hereditary condition.

One of the ways to deal with hair thinning is taking a diet rich in omega 3 fatty acids. Such foods include salmon, seeds, flax, soybeans and nuts. Also, consider using some medications that have been proven to fight hair loss and hair thinning. Some medications like finasteride and dutasteride were initially manufactured for treating prostate cancer but have also proved to be very good at remedying hair loss. Minoxidil was developed as a medication for blood pressure but is now available in medicated shampoo, spray and creams for treating hair thinning and can be bought as Rogaine.

Switching to using a high quality and effective shampoo is important as poor quality shampoos lead to hair damage and breakage. As such, don't hesitate to talk to a salon supplier or hair care specialist for advice about specialty shampoos for dealing with hair thinning especially those containing silica and biotin. It is also essential that you adopt a hairstyle which creates fullness. In this regard, we advise you to cut the hair short and then add some layers to create more volume for you thin hair. There are also many alternative treatment options that you can as well consider like acupressure, acupuncture or aromatherapy. Essential oils can also prove very helpful like rosemary, lavender, thyme and cedar wood.

You can thicken you thin hair by taking an appropriate diet especially one that contains more proteins. Experts say that a diet composed of vegetables, fruits, lean protein sources and whole grains supply the hair with essential nutrients. In addition, use of basic multivitamin supplements is also recommended as it helps in making up for nutrient deficiencies. Stress is yet another major cause of hair thinning today and in fact, this is proving to be the most serious cause of hair loss and hair thinning in modern society. Excessive worrying, surgery and illness as well as chronic anxiety all contribute greatly to hair thinning.

As such, you must learn how to deal with daily stressors through joining yoga classes, doing cardiovascular classes daily and even learning meditative practice as this will help in promoting healthy hair growth. Most importantly, do everything in your power to keep your anxieties and inner fears well balanced so that they don't cause negative physical effects to your body. Such approaches will help you cope with hair thinning and live your life to the fullest with a golden crown on your head.

5. Different Types and Patterns of Hair Loss

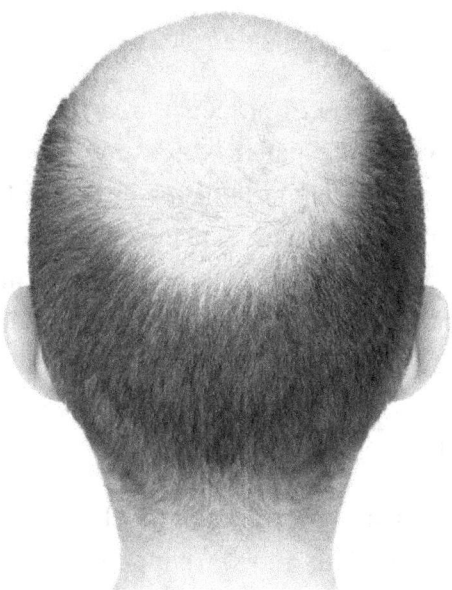

Hair loss comes in different patterns with the first one being androgenic alopecia. This type of hair loss is very common among men and women and it is also known as the male pattern baldness. It is characterized by loss or thinning of hair on head crown and receding of hair from temples. At the back and sides of the head, the hair forms a horseshoe pattern and over time, the hair can fall out completely resulting in total baldness.

Alopecia universalis is a condition involving the total loss of body and scalp hair. Alopecia totalis on the other hand denotes loss of all the scalp hair. Another condition known as alopecia areata results after the body's immune system attacks hair follicles which disrupts the normal process of hair growth and formation. While the actual cause of alopecia areata is not known, it is widely believed to be a certain form of abnormality of immune system. It is sometimes connected to autoimmune conditions like thyroid disease, allergic disorders, rheumatoid arthritis, lupus and even ulcerative colitis. This condition has been found among family members suggesting that heredity and genes also play a role in it as well.

Ophiasis is a specific type of alopecia areata where by the loss of hair happens in wave like patterns that encircles the entire head. Traction alopecia results from damages to hair follicle and papilla resulting from pulling the hair constantly or hair tension over a prolonged period of time. It is mostly present among people who tend to wear tight braids like cornrows that can lead to increased tension, break age and pulling of the hair. Additionally, hair loss can also be a result of cosmetic surgery that leads to hair tension especially facelifts.

Chignon alopecia is a type of traction alopecia where hair loss happens at the crown. This mostly happens by styling the hair in tight buns and it is very common among ballet dancers. Hypotrichosis is a condition where the hair simply doesn't grow. Unlike alopecia that involves loss of hair in areas where hair existed before, hypotrichosis represents a situation in which hair fails to grow in the first place. Another type of hair loss is telogen effluvium which happens after follicles are pushed to their resting stage prematurely by illness or stress.

Trichotillomania is a form of disorder where an individual literary pulls out his or her own hair and results in noticeable loss of hair. Lichen planopilaris disease affects the mouth and skin and can cause irritation, redness and sometimes permanent hair loss. Follicutus is a bacterial condition which leads to irritation of hair follicles through skin infection. Hairs inflicted by this condition simply fall out by themselves. Regardless of the type or pattern of hair loss you are experiencing, most of these conditions have effective conditions.

6. How to Keep Your Hair Healthy

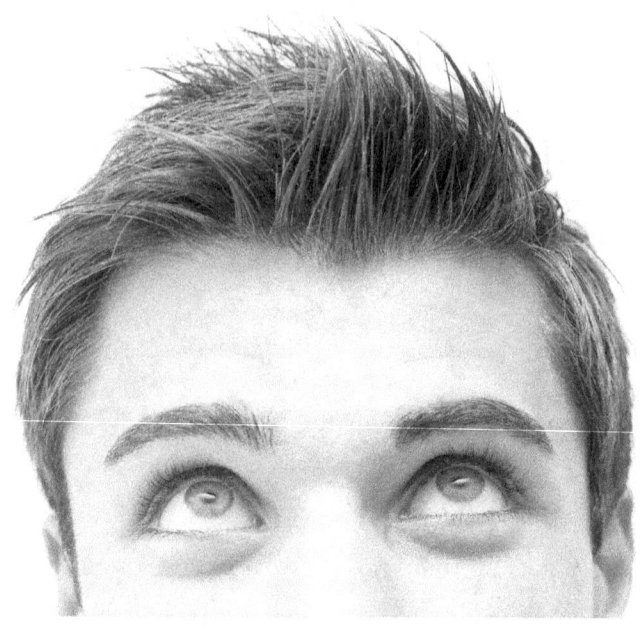

Having a vibrant, shiny and strong hair not only boosts your self esteem but also makes you confidence enough to face the world. Luckily, there are some useful tips that can help you in taking good care of your hair and ensuring that it stays healthy always. The first aspect of taking better care of your hair is washing and drying. First, you should know exactly when you need to wash your hair. Don't make the mistake of thinking that hair must be washed on a daily basis as this will cause the hair to weight down and dry out. Daily shampooing is only necessary if you have oily hair, meaning high oil production on the scalp. If you do need to shampoo every day, it's better for you to choose a lightweight shampoo. At times, washing the hair every other day can be plenty even though this will depend on your hair type.

After shampooing your hair, use a conditioner to moisturize your hair and make it soft and easily manageable. Wet hair is more vulnerable to damage unlike dry hair due to its elasticity. Due to fragility of hair when wet, using a comb with wide teeth will minimize breakage and remove tangles. Make sure that you buy conditioners and shampoo that suits the type of hair and whichever type your hair is, you will always find a specialist product that is suitable for your hair.

The other aspect of good hair care practices is use of products. First, applying hair mask encourages deep conditioning while making your hair shiny and soft.

Use serum for your hair when wet. This not only keeps your hair shiny and soft but also minimizes frizz. Actually, you just need a very small serum amount and when applying, avoid applying it on the roots as it will appear greasy. Using heat protection is important before you subject the hair to high levels of temperatures from dryers and iron. Heat is a great enemy to the hair and heat protection sprays help in locking in moisture while minimizing breakage and burning of the hair. UV shielding hair products should also be used to prevent hair damage by sun that can make your hair appear fried and lightened in color. At the same time, you should avoid products laden with chemicals especially conditioners and shampoos containing sodium chlorine, parabens or harsh sulfates. These ingredients tend to build in the hair with time and damage your locks significantly.

Eating the right food is of critical importance as far as caring for your hair is concerned. In addition to eating food rich n vitamin D and proteins which are important for strong hair, eating salmon is important as it contains the much needed omega- 3 fatty acids that are essential for healthy hair growth. Also, eat walnuts as they are known to be rich in omega 3 fatty acids, vitamin E and biotin and aids in prevention of DNA damage. Other types of foods that are essential for healthy hair growth include spinach, lentils, eggs, sweet potatoes, oysters, blueberries, poultry and vitamin supplements. Lastly, avoiding stress is not only important for your hair but stress also have serious impacts on your general health.

7. Covering and Concealing Your Hair Loss

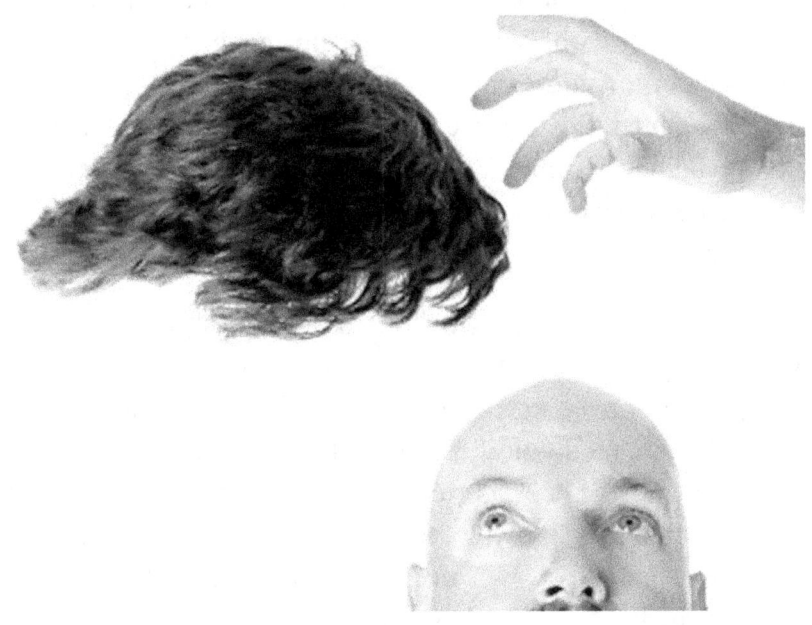

While baldness or hair loss is a reality in life, not so many people are ready or willing to admit it. Thankfully, there are many options that you can use to hide a receding hair line. First, you can decide to shave off your head, which is one of the best options for. Shaving the head can cover up a bald entirely but for women, they will definitely need to do more than this. If you are dealing with a bald, you will need to take good care of it like using sunscreen and possibly changing your shampoo.

Conceal hair loss and hair thinning with hair extensions or weaves. These are available in a wide selection and you can easily find one that suits your hair type. Try using one of the medications which boost hair re-growth. In this case, two of the most effective treatments are finasteride and Minoxidil/ Rogaine. Rogaine is an oral prescription and you just need to apply it on the scalp.

You could also consider hair transplants which involve use of surgical procedures to remove hair from other body parts and being transplanted on your bald. Additionally, don't hesitate to investigate alternative forms of surgery like scalp reduction. In this case, the bald section of your scalp is removed and remaining portions are pulled together. Scalp surgery is also highly recommended whereby the receding hairline is pulled forward. These hair transplant procedures have proved to be very effective as permanent treatments for hair loss.

Wearing a hat can conceal hair loss successfully. Unfortunately, wearing a hat is not always effective as there are times when you will of course need to remove it especially when entering an office. Nevertheless, men will do great with a hat and women can use sun hats or even wear caps as well. The market is full of many products that boost hair re- growth and you could possibly try using one of them. However, you will need to be very careful as some of the cheap remedies might end up ruining your scalp.

Wigs are very effective in concealing baldness. A wig is simply a synthetic hair piece used for covering up hair and used as a hair replacement by many. When wearing some wigs, you will need to place a translucent, thin next over the remaining hair to enable the wig fit snugly. You will also find some wigs with inner spaces that allow your natural hair to fit comfortably and use the spaces for breathing.

For smaller areas, hair loss can be concealed by using a spray which is very effective especially if you have some hair around the section for blending with. You can also try hair voluminizing products. Also, visit your clothing vendor to shop for head scarf, large sweatbands and turbans which are cost effective options to using a wig. All such options will provide you with a temporary solution to hair loss problem and you can buy some time to think about a permanent solution.

7.1 Toupee or not Toupee - Know All About Toupees

A toupee is basically a small wig that is generally worn for covering a bald spot. For many years now, toupees have been used as hair replacement alternatives, traditionally only worn by men. Most people tend to associate a toupee with poor replacement of hair and it is easy to identify a person wearing the traditional toupee is it tends to sit on the scalp unnaturally. Thankfully, significant improvements have been made on hair replacement methods and the new hair systems available on the market look completely natural and no one can spot a toupee on your head.

The best thing about using a toupee is that besides being easy to use and cost effective, the approach is non-surgical. The word 'toupee' is a French derived word that means top. For many centuries now, toupees have been used to deal with baldness and great people like Julio Caesar wore them. Later, advancements led to the toupees being redesigned to appear more natural.

Today, toupees refer to an old fashioned hair piece manufactured by injecting or knotting synthetic or human hair into the base material. Originally, a toupee was used to cover baldness but nowadays, toupees are not just used by men only but also by children and women as well experiencing hair loss. They are a sound solution for anyone experiencing hair loss problems.

You can decide to buy a ready-made toupee or simply have a custom made one to suit your specific requirements and needs. Membrane toupees are similar to small hair pieces which cover baldness and match your natural hair. They are made from a wide range of materials and different material combinations that are more comfortable, more elastic and of lighter weight for instance, a thin polyurethane material can be used for injecting hair at the base.

Using a toupee is quite beneficial. Since they are temporary hair pieces, you ready don't need to have some form of surgery performed on you. A toupee is not only important when used for hair restoration but also plays a major role in restoration of self esteem and confidence.

Before wearing a toupee, always clean and prepare the scalp properly and then attach the system. White clear liner tape should be used on polyurethane surfaces and to get the best results, you should change the tape when putting back the system. For those who don't want to replace and remove the tape now and then, a liquid hairpiece adhesive can be used to re- activate it.

Toupees also need to be cleaned regularly for better maintenance. The lace areas should be cleaned gently using a brush. The skin areas should also be scrapped off using a teaspoon to remove any residues. After cleaning and rinsing the toupee, the final step is shampooing and condition. After thoroughly rinsing the unit, a mild shampoo should be used for balancing the level of acid. Once this is done, your toupee can be reattached and you can start wearing your fresh system.

7.2 Hair Replacement Systems

Hair replacement systems are known by many names. Some people will refer to them as wigs, hairpieces and others will call them toupees. Over the years, significant improvements have been made on hair quality and materials used in construction of these hair replacement systems. For the large number of men and suffering struggling with severe hair loss, such hair systems are a great remedy to result to. However, since a hair replacement system is not your natural hair, you will need to provide them with good and regular care to sustain their natural appearance and boost your personal looks.

As usual, everyone wants to find a hair system which provides them with the most natural and unnoticeable appearance possible. In most cases, full lace hair bases can assure you this are definitely the way to go. If you are shopping for a durable hair system that will last very long, you have perfect options available such as the conventional hair base system. At other times, your need for a hair system might be more complex than just durability and appearance. You might need a system that gives you a perfect combination for durability and appearance. Maybe you even have other specific preferences like the type of hair to be used for your hair system, ventilation method or hair cut style.

Either way, there are many different bases that you can choose for a customized hair system that is perfect for you. Everyone is unique and making the best choice might appear scary. However, before making a decision, you will need to know what the bases are made from. The two materials mainly used in making hair systems are mesh fabrics and polymers. At other times, hair systems are made from a combination of these two. Polymers are used for creating imitation skin like materials that resemble the real skin tones. Polymers are highly preferred as they make durable skin systems.

Mesh fabrics on the other hand create fine lace materials and are normally made of either polyester or nylon. This material is mostly used to treat exposed base areas like front hairline.

When shopping for hair replacement systems, it is essential you ensure that you get value for what you pay for. Also, you need to shop wisely and engage yourself in comparable shopping to ensure that you get the best deals possible. As such, you will need to shop for a hair replacement system carefully and pay much attention on its quality. A good system especially a custom made one should be brand new and shouldn't be cut down in order to fit your measurements.

You should also take note of color when shopping for hair replacement systems on the internet. Your vendor should deliver a system that perfectly matches with the sample you provided. Lastly, you should look at the price of the hair replacement system to ensure that you are getting worth for your money. You can shop among several online vendors and then compare their offers to determine the most affordable deal.

7.3 Concealing Hair Loss Effectively with Hair Fibers and Powders

As another way to conceal the hair loss, many beauty care specialists and hair experts recommend use of advanced hair powders and fibers to cover the bald patches while also improving the thickness and volume of thin hair. This is the reason behind the increasing use of fibers and powders nowadays among hair loss patients.

Powders and fibers are very effective concealers not to mention that they are also totally safe. They offer an indiscernible solution to baldness and hair loss signs. They can really help your hair appear fuller and thicker in just a few seconds. The good thing with these hair loss concealers is that blend easily with the scalp and matches perfectly with the color of your hair.

Concealing hair loss with fibers cover wide areas of hair thinning and partings and since they are made with natural hair fibers, they give the user a perfect look. Applying the spray is also very easily and desirable results are delivered within the fastest time possible. By deciding to use the fibers and spray, you can easily make your thin hair appear full and thick in the safest and most natural way.

Basically, these concealers made using keratin organic fibers which immediately build the thickness and volume of the hair. The thickening hair fibers are charged electronically and can bond with hair extensions firmly which increases the volume of the hair dramatically. Thanks to them, thin hair and bald spots disappear quickly which have made them among the most preferred concealing options for bald patches among men and women.

The market has a wide range of products that can be used to conceal hair loss but what might be effective for one person might not be the best for another. These hair concealers are available in different forms ranging from hair powders and fibers to aerosol sprays and lotions. Each of these products has its pros and cons that you must consider before deciding which one to buy. Additionally, you should also consider the requirements and condition of your hair before you select any of them for trial.

For instance, sprays have been known to pose some difficulties when being applied to thinning and balding areas without seeking help. However, the best thing about the sprays is that separate applicators are not needed and the spray can cover a large bald area quickly.

After applying the thickening fiber on your scalp, the bald spots and thinned hair will start disappearing very fast. The only thing you need to do is to comb the hair and the thickened hair fibers will get fixed automatically with your natural hair strands in a manner that can't be detected. Deciding to buy hair fibers and power is the best decision you can make to conceal your hair loss and bald patches.

8. Hair Treatment and Care Options

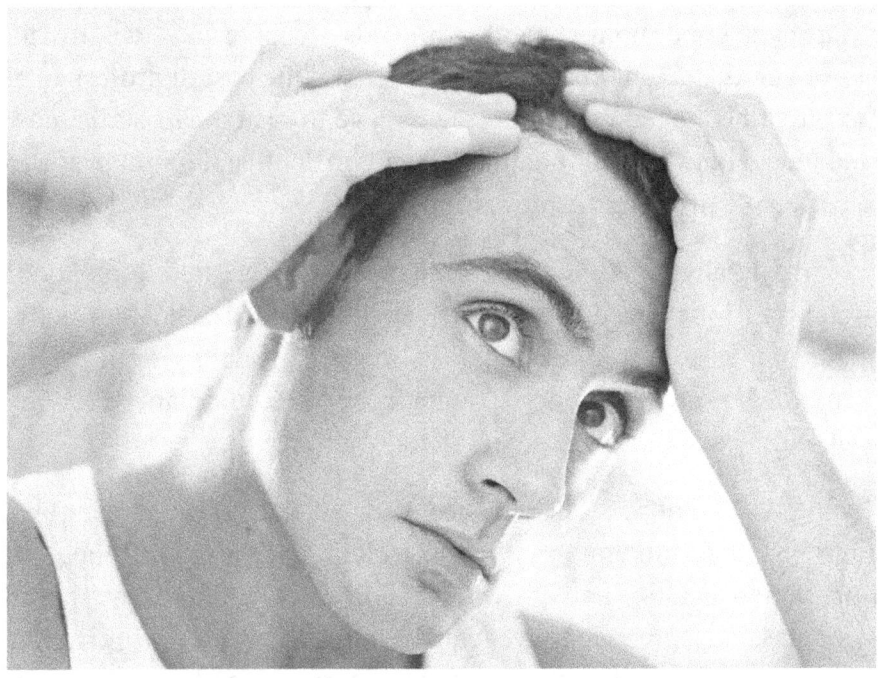

Hair loss occurs in men and women alike and there is no magical formula to cure it. However, depending on the reasons behind your loss of hair, there is a wide variety of successful treatment options available. Everyone dreams of having a beautiful, healthy and shiny hair.

While it is easy to manage and take care of short hair, most people, especially women are never contented without a thick, shiny hair. This explains why the hair fixing industry has been experiencing a boom lately. Some people think that the secret to having a well-kept, strong hair is visiting their local salons now and them.

It is essential to take good care of hair in order to avoid hair loss and other problems that can befall you. By visiting a hair salon, you will have your hair treated with oils, massages and creams which offers your hair good nourishment while also supporting its growth. However, due to our busy life schedules and the cost of professional hair treatments, not everyone can manage to visit a hair stylist now and then. Hair care and treatment is not difficult and might prove to be effective just like the professional treatment.

You might already know by now that sound sleep, taking plenty of water and a balanced diet is the secret to having a healthy body. Your hair is highly affected by your dieting habits and lifestyle. People who have improper sleeping schedules complain of having skin pimples and rashes as well as hair fall.

Eating food that is well balanced with all the essential vitamins, nutrients and minerals such as calcium and iron will help in stimulating healthy hair growth. Additionally, a good diet should contain salads, green leafy vegetables, milk and fruits. Drinking lots of water helps in boosting proper absorption and utilization of natural nutrients which promote growth of healthy hair.

The scalp needs to be massaged and moisturized on a daily basis to improve blood circulation and open pores. It is recommended that you use medicated hair oils such as thuja, jaborandi and arnica which boosts hair growth, minimizes scalp dryness and dandruffs to promote a nourished and clean scalp.

A paste of soaked fenugreek seeds and yoghurt helps in treating dandruffs which can affect growth of healthy hair. Another very effective hair conditioner is an egg especially the yolk which contains essential fatty acids, vitamins and proteins that promote healthy hair growth.

Hair care at home is an easy and simple affair and it is also very affordable compared to other hair care and treatment options. If you are suffering from excessive hair loss, you should consider consulting a reputable hair specialist so that you can have the problem treated completely.

Hair loss treatment is actually not a one-time solution but requires regular treatment so that the problem can be remedied fully and to have your hair stay healthy and shiny.

8.1 Managing Hair Loss and Thinning with Lifestyle Changes

Even though it is true that hair loss and hair thinning is a genetic condition to some extent, your lifestyle choices can affect the growth of your hair in a major way. Whether self- induced or hereditary, hair fall can be controlled easily through lifestyle change. As such, the first step towards remedying your hair loss and thinning situation is to acknowledge how your lifestyle contributes to it.

One of the common lifestyle causes of hair loss is stress. By increasing the level of cortisol in the body, prolonged stress leads to generation of excess DHT which is the main cause of male baldness or androgenetic alopecia. This kind of hair loss can only be stopped through clinically proven treatments. However, stress results in a typical non- genetic condition referred to as telogen effluvium. The condition occurs when severe or sudden levels of stress make the hair follicles to revert to a resting stage in their hair growth cycle.

While hair loss and thinning induced by stress can be corrected without using any kind of treatment, it nevertheless takes much more time. As such, you need to manage your stress levels and have some 'me- time' to reflect at your life and relax. Additionally, vigorous exercises and yoga can assist in stress alleviation and thus help you deal with your hair problems.

Smoking is another lifestyle behavior that promotes hair loss. Tobacco smoke contains toxins, carcinogens and other chemicals which damage protein molecules forming hair structure and thus retards hair growth. Besides this, smoking accelerates the process of aging besides causing hair loss, not to mention that it puts your health wellness at a great risk.

As such, it is essential that you consider changing your smoking habits so that you can minimize the kind of damage sustained on your hair. In fact, by quitting smoking, it is not only your hair that will benefit but you will also witness considerable improvement of your general health especially nails and skin.

Taking a bad diet is another lifestyle behavior that can seriously harm the healthy growth of your hair. Actually, the hair speaks a lot regarding your general health. Poor food choices lead to thinning of your hair directly. Eating disorders and iron deficiencies results in excessive loss of hair as the body diverts most of its energy towards other body areas that vitally need the energy. High sugar diets also deplete the body of essential nutrients and also impair the ability of the body to manage stress levels. If you are not getting a balanced diet by any chance, you should consider changing your diet to minimize hair loss problems.

It is important to understand that hair loss and hair thinning is not always about genes as your lifestyle has a great stake in this as well. Unfortunately some lifestyle choices and habit can deteriorate the condition of your hair. As such, maintaining a good lifestyle helps to avoid hair loss and preventing it from recurring.

8.2 The Relationship Between a Poor Diet and Hair Loss

As far as lifestyle is concerned, dieting can have a great impact on your hair growth. To be more precise, a poor diet causes hair thinning and hair loss.

A good diet promotes the building of hair structure which can make the hair to stay healthy easily. To prevent loss of hair, you should take foods that contain essential nutrients. Hair basically has a very simple structure. The roots enable the hair to stay in place on your head. The outer layer comprises of the cuticle which protects inner hair parts and also regulates the content of moisture in the hair fibers. Middle layer or cortex contains hair color as well as other special qualities of the hair like elasticity and curls.

When you fail to supply your body with sufficient nutrients, the body results in distributing the limited nutrients supply to parts of the body that really need them. The list of the vital parts includes lungs and heart among others. Since hair is not a part of them, it will receive little to no nutrients and this result in hair loss.

The hair fails to receive enough nourishment due to nutrition deficiencies, unbalanced diets, taking plenty of fast foods and poverty among other factors. Failure to get enough nutrition increases hair shedding and this can also damage the hair shafts which seriously retards hair growth and re-growth.

There are some nutrients that can ultimately lead to loss of hair if they are not present in food. For instance, proteins are critical for muscle building and are also needed by all cells and tissues in the body including hair. As such, hair will only grow normally if you take a diet rich in nutrients. Vitamins are also needed for effective hair growth especially vitamin A, B6, B12 and Vitamin C. Most importantly, vitamins help in preventing hair breakage or splitting.

Going by the above illustrations, it is pretty clear that there is a very strong connection between hair loss and a poor diet. If you have a poor diet, you can rest assured that your hair will start falling out. However, this is not hair loss as it is caused by nutrition deficiencies. The most critical nutrients needed for healthy hair growth are vitamins and proteins. As such, it is advisable that your food contains certain types of foods such as leafy green leaves, oyster, eggs, blueberries, nuts and yoghurt among other foods to boost your hair.

Following a poor diet puts your hair in a serious risk and minimizes your chances of having a beautiful, healthy hair. By including some of these essential nutrients in your menu, it is easy to prevent loss of hair and improve your overall healthiness.

8.3 Supplements for Hair Loss Treatment

The process of natural hair cycle involves between 50 and 150 hairs falling a day. Actually, this cycle of hair loss is quite normal as 90 percent of the hair is in its growth stage while the rest is resting. The normal cycle of hair re-growth takes an estimated period of between 2 and 3 years. After all the resting hair has fallen out completely, new hair tends to grow after between 3 and 4 months.

Unfortunately, due to some factors such as age and lifestyle, people lose more in a day than the average 50-100 hair falls. When you realize that the natural hair loss process has become excessive, it is necessary that you take the right measures to minimize the fall. Fortunately, the market is a hub of multiple hair loss medications and products. In the recent years, hair loss supplements have become quite popular especially among people looking for a hair balding product. The reason why most of these supplements are very effective in containing hair loss is that they are manufactured using natural ingredients which are very effective in inhibition of balding process.

Natural hair thinning supplements are manufactured through a formulation of natural ingredients including zinc, minerals, vitamins and amino acids. Other ingredients that you should look for in the product are such as saw palmetto, bay root and nettle, grape seed extract, bay/ lavender essential oils and pygeum extract. Most of these ingredients are known to inhibit production of DHT hormone naturally which is the major cause of balding and hair loss in men. Some of the most effective hair loss supplements include viviscal, nioxin, hairomega, HairTopia, Procerin, Hair Formula 37, Melanchor and Nexxus Vita Tress among others. Another natural remedy that can deal with hair loss and thinning is meditation. It restores hormonal balance and reduces stress.

Procerin is one of the most remarkable hair supplements out there with tests showing that it has a success rate of 88 percent. It has received great reviews from consumers not just for its fantastic results only but it is also sold in an affordable price as well. Currently, it is one of most effective herbal hair growth supplements on the market. Another supplement is Hair Genesis, a botanically derived supplement that is designed to stop hair loss and promote re- growth. The oral supplement blocks DHT from progressing, attacking and damage hair follicles which could lead to permanent hair loss.

Profollica has received satisfactory ratings from its users. This hair re-growth formulation is specifically designed to treat androgenetic alopecia which is the major cause for the male pattern hair loss. Propecia boasts of being the only prescription/ supplement medication to be approved by FDA for treating male pattern baldness. The supplement has recorded a success rate of about 66 percent even though it has been largely associated with some sexual side effects.

Overall, most of the hair loss supplements out there give impressive results but as always, choosing a supplement is a personal choice and you should be well informed when choosing yours.

8.4 Hair Laser Therapeutic Treatment

Hair laser therapeutic treatment is one of the options available for stopping hair loss. Basically, effective hair loss treatments are those that address underlying hair loss causes which it is designed to tackle. Even though it is widely believed that loss of hair especially among men is a natural process facilitated by genetic factors, recent researches have shown that a wide range of factors are involved. As such, hair loss could be triggered or accelerated by hormones, stress, medicine side effects, nutrient deficiencies and tight scalp among other factors.

Hormones also have a huge role to play in hair loss as they affect hair follicles. Estrogens and androgens are female and male hormones in the body and correcting their imbalance helps to treat hair loss effectively. However, hair laser therapy has distinguished itself as one of the most successful treatments for hair loss. It is one of the most recent innovative developments in the world of medical technology. It is a non invasive, non chemical and a non surgical scientific procedure within cosmetic treatment for scalp problems, hair thinning and hair loss. The solution has been proved and tested clinically and found to be efficient and harmless and with no any side effects noted.

A new research found that laser hair therapy stops hair loss with a success rate of 85 percent and promotes hair re-growth by 55 percent. Those who have tried this therapy have noted that they feel and look fuller and stronger in their heads and their hair gets much healthier. Laser therapeutic procedure stimulates growth of hair in two ways. First, the use of coherent light energy during the laser procedure leads to the transfer of energy to hair follicles in a similar way in which light assists a plant to grow.

Additionally, the light improves and stimulates circulation of blood around hair follicles and thus flushes away DHT. This leads to the growing back of fuller and thicker hair after the treatment. However, laser therapeutic is in no way a magical cure and just like Propecia and Minoxidil, people respond to the treatment differently. Most women and men who decided to give laser treatment a chance have enjoyed positive changes. The good thing with laser hair technology is that it causes no thermal, pain or damage. The process involves absolutely no burning sensation or cutting and works with soft laser that utilizes much less energy even than the normal 40- watt light bulb.

Laser lights penetrate into the skin easily and can help in successfully dealing with hair loss. It is one of the most successful and safest hair loss treatments in modern world and you should definitely include it in your hair re-grow strategy. Considering that the best way to deal with hair loss is to boost supply of blood in the hair follicles and scalp, laser hair is able to do exactly that which explains its incredibly amazing results. Boosting blood circulation promotes supply of essential nutrients and even oxygen to hair follicles and flushing our detrimental wastes like DHT.

8.5 Topical Treatments

Medical researchers are yet to find a cure that can treat baldness completely. However, topical hair loss treatments like some scalp treatments and special shampoos can effectively complement other proven treatments like Rogaine, surgical hair restoration and Propecia. Unfortunately, most of the claims and promises given by most of the topical treatments for hair loss are not completely proven. As such, when shopping for any topical treatment, you should be well informed about its effectiveness and whether it offers you value for money or not.

DHT blockers are perhaps the most popular topical treatments and they work by inhibiting loss of hair at its roots. Most of the DHT blockers out there claim that they are able to minimize amount of DHT available in your scalp and thus control hair loss. Even though some people have used them, their success rate is yet to be proved clinically. However, considering that DHT is one of the major causes of hair loss, it is highly likely that any topical treatment that can successfully block DHT can go a long way in providing a solution to the hair loss problem.

Another topical treatment is Revivogen. According to its manufacturer, this topical treatment successfully inhibits 5-alpha reductase enzyme that is responsible for conversion of testosterone to DHT. Going by this, it is undeniable that Revivogen is one of the most effective topical treatments out there on the market. Crinagen is yet another topical treatment. Manufactured as a spray, the popularity of Crinagen lies on the fact that it is completely natural thus very safe on the body. Additionally, the treatment doesn't have any alcohol and there are no undesirable side effects associated with it. It is equally effective and safe for both men and women. The most important ingredients in the product are azelaic acid and Proanthocyanidins which nourish hair follicles and reduce the amount of DHT in the scalp.

Hair growth stimulators are mostly used to relieve thinning hair rather than promoting hair re- growth. They contain some very effective ingredients such as Folligen, Tricomin, Retin- A, Nano Shampoo, Prox- N and Proxiphen. Tricomin is another treatment used by both mean and women. This spray has been tested scientifically and found to be very beneficial for hair growth and development. Besides the spray, you can also find Tricomin in for conditioners and shampoos.

Shampoos and conditioners have always been at the front line in the fight against hair loss. However, these two treatments can cause some undesirable side effects which can at times increase loss of hair when left uncontrolled. Nizoral is a shampoo that has been found to fit with a wide range of treatment options. Made for both men and women, Nozoral is very effective in reducing inflammation and itching caused by other hair loss treatments like Propecia. Additionally, this shampoo promotes scalp health and can help to treat both female and male pattern baldness.

Lastly, Nioxin shampoo and conditioners are effective topical treatments for dealing with thinning or fine hair.

8.6 Hair Loss Shampoo Guidelines

Many people are not sure about the best care options for their scalp and hair. Hair loss shampoo is undeniably the most common solution for hair loss.

As you might already know, a hair loss shampoo is a kind of cleansing agent which contains chemicals such as sodium lauryl sulfate. These chemicals help in removal of unwanted build ups in the scalp and hair, keeping them manageable and clean. If you buy a shampoo, you will realize that it has been designed to deal with three major hair conditions. These are dry hair, oily hair and normal hair. What makes the shampoos different is amount of the hair moisturizing oil contained in them. For instance, a shampoo made for dry hair contains the highest amount of hair moisturizing oil since it is supposed to ensure that the hair doesn't stay in its dried state after being washed.

Buying the right shampoo for your hair is very important. Just a simple mistake of using the wrong shampoo for your specific hair condition might compromise the health of the hair and cause hair loss and thinning in the long run. In addition to having different types of shampoos, they are also divided depending on the level of PH they contain. Since shampoos are made using chemicals, they are naturally alkaline which makes the hair to tangle easily. To counter this effect, manufacturers have produced PH balanced and acidic shampoos.

Another group of shampoos comprise of those containing special medicated ingredients that are extracted from natural plants or herbs. These shampoos are very effective when used to treat scalp problems like itchiness and dandruff. While it is true that these herbal shampoos are very beneficial in maintaining healthiness of the hair, the truth is that they are of little effectiveness when used to deal with loss of hair. This is unless you consider using special shampoos for hair loss like DHT blocker shampoo.

Normal shampoos can still prevent temporary loss of hair and improve the condition of the scalp as well. However, such results can only be achieved by using the proper type of shampoos regularly and in the best way possible. This will help in keeping your scalp and hair clean and removing off toxins like androgen that lead to hair loss. People make some serious mistakes when using shampoos such as pouring in on the scalp directly when washing. This will clean the hair unevenly. As such, you should lather you shampoo on the palm and scrub it gently using some moderate strength and then rinse off your hair thoroughly.

The only way to be guaranteed of the best results is by buying the right shampoo for your hair condition and using it appropriately. This will guarantee that your hair stays in its healthiest condition for many years to come.

9. Slowing Down Hair Loss

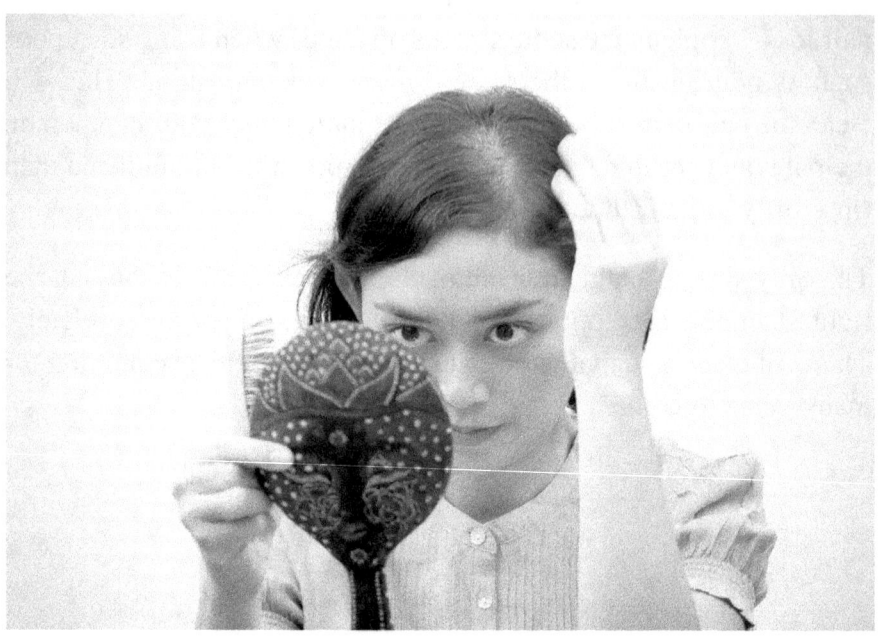

Hair is a crowning glory for human beings. Unless you are the kind of person who regards a bald to being a fashion statement, people don't take the issue of hair loss kindly let alone being bald. Thankfully, there are so many ways in which you can slow down hair loss and age gracefully with your hair still being intact on your head.

To start with, most people have no idea that caffeine can help to slow down hair loss. However, research has shown that caffeine is effective in dealing with female baldness. Basically, caffeine decreases the amount of DHT on the scalp which is known to cause structural damage to hair follicles. Caffeine, obtained in either tea or coffee, will not only slow down hair loss but also helps in easing mood swings and stress. Next, lean protein helps to decelerate hair loss and it is found mostly in the skinless poultry. It acts as a perfect source for the lean protein which is rich in zinc and iron. It is widely known that deficiency of zinc and iron in the body triggers hair loss. Since hair mostly comprises of keratin, it therefore requires proteins for the hair to stay healthy and strong.

It is also advisable that you eat plenty of veggies such as carrots and cauliflower to reduce hair loss. Vegetables are known to be a perfect source of vitamins, especially B6, biotin and foliate that not only slows down loss of hair but also promotes growth of hair on the scalp. Next, shampoos are good for hair care and maintenance but most importantly, it is advisable that you use the right type of shampoo depending on your hair type and condition. You should beware of shampoos containing sodium Lauryl Sulfate or sodium laureth sulfate as both of these are actually degreasing agents which alleviate oil and dirt.

The problem of this particular chemical additive is that it can cause hair thinning when used for a long period of time. As such, using a natural shampoo can really help in reducing hair loss especially those that are 100% herbal. Most importantly, search for shampoos containing saw palmetto, green tea and aloe Vera. Green tea shampoos are not only effectively but are also very affordable as well.

Even though foods are very useful in promoting growth of hair and minimizing hair loss, proper hair care and maintenance is very essential. Most importantly, be very careful about products that you use on your hair and avoid those containing alcohol like gels. These products strip the hair of essential natural oils which keeps the hair strong and prevents breakages. Also, it is essential that you brush the hair gently. Vigorous hair brushing can make hair strands to break. Also, rubbing the hair during towel drying causes further breakage and should be avoided. If your hair still continues to fall even after trying out these options, it is essential that you visit your doctor for professional advice and treatment.

9.1 How to Prevent or Reduce Hair Loss

Most sufferers of hair loss grow more nervous, scared and nervous every day. Finding out that you are losing a lot of hair on the pillow or comb can make you feel very much frustrated. In this regard, you should learn about the best ways to prevent and reduce loss of hair to ensure that it doesn't control and consume you. First, the most important thing is to find out the exact cause of your hair loss. This can be caused by many factors ranging from stress, diet, fungal and bacterial infections, diabetes, pregnancy and trauma among other factors.

The good thing with the above causes is that they only cause temporary hair loss which can be controlled easily. If you are one of those people who suffer from hair loss related to hormones or genes, there are still some ways that you can keep the problem in control and minimize the rate of hair loss significantly. The first milestone in taking good care of your hair and minimizing the loss is by taking a proper diet and exercising a lot. Hair contains some protein that it requires to maintain and build hair follicles. As such, getting sufficient proteins will keep your follicles and scalp healthy and reduce the rate of loss.

Exercising boosts circulation of blood to the scalp and entire body. This helps in ensuring that the roots are properly nourished. Trying to reduce your anxiety and stress levels will help reduce hair loss significantly as well. Stress leads to the tightening up of body muscles which inhibits proper circulation of blood. As such, anything that can help alleviate your stress levels ranging from exercising and meditation to taking breaks and going for yoga classes will help prevent hair loss in major ways.

Being kind to your hair always will also prevent its loss. For instance, avoid washing your hair with harsh chemicals as they will not only make it dry but will also damage hair follicles. Treating your hair chemically will also cause thinning and will strip the hair of its proteins and nutrients. On the same note, it is also essential that you minimize your use of curlers, blow dryers and hair irons as this will keep your hair and scalp healthy.

The market is a hub of so many products which claim to be very effective in preventing and reducing hair loss. However, it is important that you investigate and experiment extensively first before endorsing any of them. This will help avoid using products that can pose serious risks on your hair. Most people have also used natural remedies successfully to prevent hair loss. Some of them like essential oils, herbal solutions and saw palmetto are some of the best natural remedies that you can use for your hair. You can buy them at nutrition and health stores on the internet.

Always remember to experiment with different hair products until you find one that works best for your hair. This will help in preventing hair loss and hair thinning.

9.2 Hair Loss Diet Supplements

Diet supplements are considered to be effective in promoting hair growth. They provide the body with the necessary nutrients so that the hair grows healthily and prevent hair fall.

One of the commonly used diet supplements for fighting hair loss is PABA which is one of the B vitamins. Its main role in promoting hair health is that it acts as an effective and very beneficial anti graying supplement. According to recent researches undertaken, people who take low PABA diets are highly likely to have gray hair. However, increasing your PABA intake restores your normal hair color almost immediately. In line with deficiency of Folic Acid, Biotin and Pantothenic Acid, lack of PABA in your diet will definitely impact negatively on your hair color and quality. Liver is the best source of PABA even though it is also available in kidneys, whole grain and yeast.

Another very important hair loss supplement is inositol, one of the B vitamins. This compound naturally occurs in the liver, eyes, muscles, brain and the kidney. Consuming a diet that lacks inositol can lead to formation of bald spots. In fact, lack of inositol has more serious hair loss effects more in males than females. In addition, the compound has other benefits besides promoting hair growth such as lowering high blood pressure. Vitamin supplements have been known to be very effective in dealing with hair loss and scalp issues.

B family vitamin supplements are perhaps the most important in fighting hair loss and inadequacy of B6, folic acid and insotil can accelerate the process of hair fall. Even though most of these vitamins are readily available in a wide variety of foods containing beta carotene as well as orange juice, it is very unfortunate that most people do not get sufficient B vitamins from their diet. As such, vitamin supplements that are rich in these vitamin B complexes can be the ultimate solution for your hair loss problem.

Besides vitamin B complex, there are other minerals that are very effective in preventing loss of hair. A recent research showed that rats fed with a magnesium deficient diet lost hair in clumps which could be a similar scenario in human beings as well. However, the researchers also realized that the condition is reversible after satisfying the deficiency. Unfortunately, the same researchers have also founded that excessive exposure some vitamins might encourage loss of hair.

For instance, taking vitamin A excessively might trigger hair loss and thinning. Some vitamin supplements not only prevent loss of hair but also maintain the hair in its perfect condition. Vitamin C for example promotes circulation of blood in the scalp which minimizes the chances of hair falling out. In summary, it is very clear that diet supplements can help in reversing and stopping hair loss successfully.

9.3 Top Prescription Medications for Hair Loss

There are so many shampoos and medications that can help in dealing with hair loss problem. However, most of these products do not have solid scientific proof. Minoxidil and Finasteride are the only two prescription medications for hair loss that are approved by drug authorities. Most of the topical hair products available on the market today contain these two elements and most customers have also attested to the effectiveness of having them in the medications.

Despite the effectiveness of some prescription medications for hair loss, they also enjoy some criticisms as well. For instance, some users have complained that these products only have short lived results and meaningful results are only seen only when they are in use. Nonetheless, Minoxidil and Finasteride have been a great aid to people with hair loss issues. One of the most popular products for treating hair loss is Rogaine, a drug known to be a vasodilator. As such, Rogaine promotes dilation of blood vessels when applied on the scalp regularly. Researchers have ascertained that Rogaine is very effective in preventing loss of hair especially on the crown.

Loniten is another prescription medication containing Minoxidil and the prescription drug is available as a pill. Initially, Loniten was designed to help in lowering blood pressure and researchers have discovered that one of its side effects is promoting hair growth. Unfortunately, this medication also has some undesirable side effects on the user like breathing difficulties, issues of drug interaction, water retention and an increase in heart rate. Another product worth mentioning is EXT Extreme Hair Therapy which has enjoyed increased popularity thanks to its effectiveness in dealing with hair loss.

As far as Finasteride products are concerned, one of the most renowned products in this category is Propecia. Just like Loniten, it was not originally manufactured to treat loss of hair. Promoted as Proscar initially, this medication was used to treat enlarged prostate among men. It was later realized that it promoted hair growth as one of its side effects and thus led to the introduction of Propecia. Besides, slowing the rate of hair loss in men, the product has also proved to be very effective when used to treat baldness. Unfortunately, just like any other prescription medications, Propecia comes with its share of undesirable health effects.

Surprisingly, most of these products have proved to be very effective in promoting hair re- growth. They help in promoting growth of healthy hair back on the scalp. Even though these medications won't manage in making hair to grow back and fill your entire, they successfully slow down the rate of hair loss. You can use them to fill some of your pronounced areas. Nonetheless, medical scientists and researchers have been working hard to discover and testing hair loss solutions and this will soon lead to discovery of prescription medications with minimal unwanted side effects.

9.4 A Look at Low-Level Laser Therapy

Low level laser therapy is a recently discovered interesting procedure for treating hair loss. This non- surgical treatment alternative has proved quite effective in treatment of chronic pain, aiding in wound healing decreasing inflammation. Otherwise abbreviated as LLLT, new discoveries show that it can easily induce hair growth. When investigating whether LLLT can actually cause cancer or not in mice, a Hungarian researcher realized that spots treated depicted an increase in hair growth. An observation made in 1960's, it was not until recently that researchers have re-visited the issue more seriously.

Ideally, doctors don't have a very clear explanation on exactly how LLLT actually promotes growth of hair. According to one theory pioneered by the doctors, it is believed that low level laser technology increases circulation of blood on the treated area. There is still another theory suggesting that LLLT successfully transfer light energy to hair cells directly which leads to increased growth activity as energy is available in abundance. However, this technology doesn't seem to work on other areas that are bald completely. Also, for the effects to be maintained, the treatment needs constant maintenance.

Devices used in low level laser technology are available in two major varieties. There are those that are specifically designed for use at the doctor's office and those that hair loss patients can use at home. Home devices enable the user to perform laser treatment at the comfort of their home. However, as you would expect, these devices do not provide as much intensity and coverage like the systems based at the doctor's office. Even though doctor's devices come with the benefit of greater coverage and energy, best results are only achieve by undertaking repeated trips to doctor's office to have the treatment performed. There are no studies yet to show which of the two devices the better one is.

While there are so many LLLT home devices available out there on the market, the only device approved for being effective in treating loss of hair is Hairmax Lasercomb. This device is very effective for promoting hair growth among males suffering from Androgenetic Alopecia. Low level laser technology is truly very effective in dealing with androgenic alopecia in both males and females. However, doctors also say that this treatment doesn't show any signs of effectiveness when used on areas that already bald. It is much more useful when used on areas experiencing hair thinning.

Rather than treating yourself at home, it is advisable that you get treatment at a physician's office for best results. Treatment protocol in a typical office involves going for regular treatments, about 2 or 3 times in a week at least for 6 weeks. Then, for the next 3 or 4 months, you can go for treatment once in a week. In case low level laser technology delivers positive results, you should also consider going for additional procedures and touch up. As such, it is essential that you give LLLT a chance when thinking about an effective hair loss prevention regime.

9.5 Topical Hair Loss Treatment Varieties

Another popular options to consider are topical hair loss treatments. This classification also has several varieties that you should know about when deciding about the best hair loss treatment to use.

The first topical treatment includes the anti- inflammatories that are very effective in dealing with numerous hair problems such as flaking, itching, inflammation and redness. Some experts will advocate for use of a diet rich in vegetables and with low levels of refined carbohydrates and bad fats. Such a diet is a good alternative in reducing inflammation in the body.

Another topical treatment is Azelaic acid which is a highly effective ingredient present in numerous types of topical hair loss treatments. Azelaic acid hinders formation of DHT on scalp. The acid is found naturally in various substances such as barley, wheat and rye and has also been found to be very effective when used to treat certain skin disorders.

Concealers are very common in the world of hair loss and include various treatments that can be applied on the scalp directly. These substances amazingly reduce appearance of hair loss patches and baldness on the head. Additionally, they boost fullness of thinning hairs while also reducing the contrast that exists between thinning locks and balding scalp. DHT blockers are also very effective topical treatments that can cure a variety of hair problems. Just as their name suggest, DHT blockers reduce the amount of DHT contained in the scalp and leads to hair loss. These DHT Blockers can be applied on the scalp directly.

Growth stimulators function by boosting hair growth and stimulating re-growth of hair. However, it is essential to understand that growth simulators do not actually stop hair from falling largely because they don't deal with the core causes of hair loss. As such, it is advisable that you use these growth stimulators just to supplement other topical treatments and not using them as the main treatment.

Nettle root extract is an active ingredient obtained from stinging nettle plant. Besides being used as a hair treatment, people have used nettle root extract all over the world as an addition in soups and salads as it adds flavor. Superoxide dismutase is another very effective topical treatment when it comes to stopping hair fall. The product works by lowering super oxide levels in the body and promote hair growth at the same time.

Topical treatments are placed on the scalp directly unlike surgery or pills. They are available in different forms including conditioners, shampoos and creams. Rogaine is a very popular hair loss topical treatment that is used by both men and women alike. Additionally, there are other topical products that contain Minoxidil and are very effective when it comes to cleansing the scalp and removing dead skin that builds up and accumulates on the scalp. You can purchase any of your favorite topical treatment on the internet and enjoy fast hair restoration and re-growth.

10. Natural Hair Loss Treatments

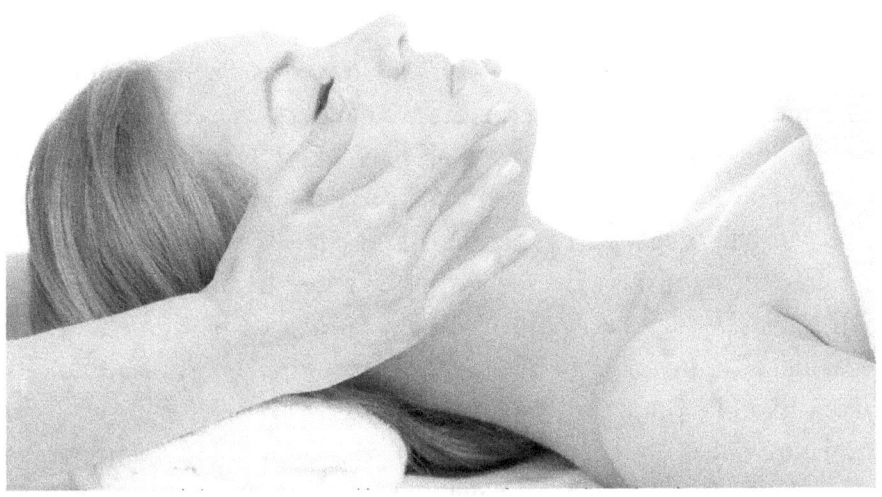

Although they have not been scientifically proven, there are many natural treatment options available. Depending on the cause of hair loss, some methods are reported effective in treating hair loss. You can make the natural treatment at your home or simply buy over the counter.

Just like other products, the effectiveness of these treatments varies a lot but you have a wide range of options to select from. Dry Alma and Coconut Oil is highly recommended for stimulating the hair and can reduce loss of hair significantly. To use this product, you need to prepare a tonic by mixing the coconut oil with the dry Alma and gently applying it on your scalp.

Another highly effective natural hair loss treatment that you should consider is olive oil for cleansing your hair strands. Home-made olive oil is a very effective treatment for thinning hair. Besides providing your scalp and hair with the essential proteins needed for growth, the treatment also penetrates in the scalp and removes dirt clogging in the hair follicles. Such clogged follicles interfere with the ability of the hair to absorb nutrients better and results in hair thinning.

Herbs and supplements are a core treatment as far as natural hair loss medications are concerned. Saw palmetto is very effective in promoting healthy hair growth as it blocks DHT production that causes hair loss. Adding vitamin to your eating regime also reduces loss of hair especially vitamin A, E and B vitamins. Topical treatments are also very essential in hair loss treatments especially when massaging the scalp. Use some drops of bay essential oil, sesame oil or lavender to massage the base of the scalp. Natural oils like olive oil, canola oil and safflower are very useful in restoring moisture. Also, try rubbing the scalp with ginger juice, onion juice or garlic juice to boost hair growth. Other natural treatments include green tea, rangoli henna and boiling rosemary and potatoes in water and applying it on your hair.

Lifestyle changes are also a key aspect of natural hair loss treatments. This includes adding more proteins in your diet like fish, lean meats, soy and fish. Also, it is paramount that you take good care of your hair such as not brushing it when wet and applying the right hair treatment products. Reducing stress is important as it is a major cause of hair loss. This requires that you practice meditation, do some exercises by walking, swimming or biking and talking or writing about it.

If you opt to buy natural treatments from over the counter, there are certain factors that you should consider. First, choose products containing approved ingredients as others might harm your hair. Most importantly, consider buying a natural treatment with Minoxidil as an ingredient as it plays a major role in enhancing hair growth. It contains essential amino acids which are needed to boost natural hair growth. Next, consider buying products with easily understandable instructions. Just like other treatments, you can only get the best results by following the guidelines to the letter. Some of these treatments require that they be used regularly and be applied on the hair several times in a day. If you manage to select the right natural treatment for your hair, you will never have to worry about hair loss and thinning any more.

10.1 Natural Hair Loss Treatment Tips for Women

Women become disturbed a lot when their precious, long strands start to fall and become thinner and thinner day by day. When this happens, it is essential that you confront the problem as soon as possible before it is too late. However, many women do not realize that going natural might be the solution for their woes. The natural treatments help you avoid wasting your time and money on painful surgical procedures and using commercial products.

The main reason why a lot of women opt to use natural hair loss treatments is because they are much safer unlike most of the artificial hair treatments. In fact, most women will consider using natural treatments first and only revert to using commercial products once they realize that the natural treatments are not effective. The first aspect of natural hair loss treatment for women involves reviving your hair follicles in order to boost hair growth. This can be done by taking more folic acids as using these vitamins constantly helps in minimizing hair fall. Livening up your diet also helps in boosting hair growth and reducing hair thinning. For starters, eat more organic foods and opt for foods that are rich in sulfur, magnesium and zinc. Also, increase your intake for vitamins especially vitamin A, D, E and B5. Also, increase your intake for herbal supplements by taking rosemary and sage and incorporate ginger and garlic in your meals. Drinking more green tea will also help.

Vitamins are an essential natural hair loss treatment for women. Vitamin A can be obtained from fish, peas and nuts which promote growth of shinier and smoother hair. Niacin or vitamin B3 is essential in promoting fast hair growth. Hair loss and thinning in women is largely attributed to poor absorption of nutrients which can result from insufficient amount of acid in the stomach. As such taking hydrochloric acid tablets can stimulate hair re-growth. Other treatments that can help are such as applying jojoba oil, kalaya oil/ emu oil and arnica on the scalp. In addition, sage, safflower and rosemary are also very useful in enhancing hair growth when applied on the scalp.

Next, water is an essential aspect for good health and drinking plenty of water daily will go a long way in saving your hair. Make sure you take a minimum of 8 glasses in a day to boost circulation of blood in your body. Hair follicles and scalp benefit a lot from efficient blood circulation as water flushes out toxins that could be hindering your hair growth. Additionally, if you choose to treat loss of hair naturally, taking a proper and balanced diet plan is a must. Hair thinning and hair loss are mostly caused by hormonal imbalance that can be brought about by eating the wrong food types. Most importantly, focus more on eating healthy foods while minimizing sweet and junky food that can easily compromise your health wellness.

Use of vitamin supplements is an essential part of natural hair loss treatment regime especially those that are rich in B Vitamins and vitamin A, C and E. Biotin and Inositol vitamins helps in promoting effective and safe hair growth. As such, use of vitamin supplements makes a lot of sense especially for women experiencing vitamin deficiency. There is also a wide range of herbal remedies that you can use to combat natural hair loss. For instance, taking a cup of rosemary teal will help you combat the hair loss problem. Other herbs that are essential in treatment of hair loss are ginseng, saw palmetto and nettle roots.

If you try the above options and tips before buying commercial hair treatments, you will enjoy an effective, safe and low cost natural hair loss treatment.

10.2 Learn How to Handle Stress the Best Way

It is well known that people pull out their hair willfully when anxious but it is also a fact that chronic stress also results in inadvertent loss of hair. Physiological changes caused by intense and frequent stressors have a huge impact on hair loss. When people are faced with powerful stressors, like illness or a life changing events such as divorce or childbirth, most of the hair goes into a resting pace and within a few months, the hair starts to fall. According to doctors, stress related hair loss is just a way in which the body takes some time as it prepares itself to address large problems like coping with the stressor or recovery.

Some of the most common physiological stressors linked to loss of hair include caloric deficiency, hormone fluctuations especially in women as well as fast weight gain/loss. When faced with loneliness, anxiety, stress, tension, frustration and fatigue, people also tend to pull off hair from their head. Severe stress can lead to hair follicles being attacked by the white blood cells that stopping growth of hair and leading to its fall out.

Stress manifests itself in various ways and in different situations in life. It is also influenced by a wide range of factors such as age, family upbringing, education, spouse, friends and environment alongside other society relations you have. Unfortunately, stress has very serious effects on your health and showcases itself in numerous such as appearance of wrinkles and fine lines as well as hair loss and other health effects. Stress is present among adults and children as well. It is this very important that you learn about the best strategies of handling stress in order to live a happy and fruitful life.

Even though stress levels can be frightful, huge and unbearable at times, you must have the faith and stamina of handling it and taking charge of your life. Hidden stress can easily cause headaches, sleeplessness, tintinnus and other serious health effects. You should thus beware of constructive ways of alleviating stress like increasing your consumption of foods rich in Vitamin C such as juices or fruits, drink dark tea as it contains flavonoids that help in fighting stress and eat pistachios to regulate blood supply in the body. Eating strawberries will also keep you calm and help you fight stress in style.

People sometimes use certain strategies to help them reduce stress temporarily but what they don't understand is that these strategies could lead to more damages in the long run. As such, some behaviors like drinking, smoking, under eating or overeating, withdrawing from family and friends, using relaxation drugs ad pills, sleeping too much to escape stressors and procrastinating will only end up causing more harm rather than helping you solve the problem. Also, taking out your high stress levels on others through physical violence, angry outbursts and lashing out will not help.

A good strategy to handle stress is to change how you think. Your thinking has profound impacts on your physical and emotional well being. When you think negatively, the body reacts as if it is in a tension situation. Thinking positively makes the body to release chemicals which contribute to making you feel great about you and relaxed. You should also work hard to eliminate certain words from your vocabulary such as 'always', 'must', 'should' and 'never'. Such definitive statements will only end up creating stress as they are self defeating on your body. Learn to live a life where you don't force yourself to control things you have no control.

Most people experience stress due to poor time management skills. If you learn how to manage your limited time better and more effectively, you can as well forget about stress. Most importantly, avoid multitasking regardless of how good you think you are as the human mind is created to handle one thing at a time. Lastly, learn to keep your life as simplest as possible and teach yourself to say no. Making your life complicated will give you a feeling as if life is running out of you.

10.3 How Quality of Sleep Contributes to Hair Loss

You will never realize how important your hair is until it starts to leave you and the idea of going bald dawns on you. When hair starts thinning out and falling like dry leaves during autumn, you start to panic and you are determined to pay any cost just to see hair grow back on your head. However, what most people fail to realize that most of the culprits in hair loss are the simple things that we do. Unknowingly to many, the quality of sleep has a great impact on hair loss as you shall soon find out here below.

Once you fail to get a good night's sleep, the body is unable to rejuvenate and restore itself. It thus fails to rebuild its cells which keep it string. When this happens, the body gets in a desperate state as it starts to search for proteins so that that it can naturally restore itself and make up for lack of rest. The best sources of proteins in the body include the skin, nails and hair. If you have bad hair, chances are also high that your skin and nails are also bad as well. While the fix certainly can't happen overnight, you can change things slowly by slowly by ensuring that you have a sound night's sleep. Over time, you will start to notice remarkable changes on your hair.

Having a good sleep quality prevents the body from restoring itself with your hair. When this happens, you simply end up losing your hair. The best secret is to go sleep early so that you can be able to wake up early the next day. The body also loves to sleep in a completely dark and quite environment. As such, make sure that you sleep in a place where you are not disturbed by sounds regardless of how tiny they are. Even though there is no so much scientific evidence on exactly why a human body needs to sleep, it is an undeniable fact that sleep is crucial for optimal health, growth and development.

The only unfortunate thing is that most people in the modern world are so much willing to deprive themselves of sleep. When it comes to meeting the many demands in our life, most people won't think twice about sacrificing their sleep and have no idea of the kind of harm they expose themselves to. Researchers have reported that sleep deprivation, regardless of how small it is, can have a significant effect on your health, productivity, cognitive capacity and mood. By having enough sleep, you tend to become more focused and you generally feel great about yourself.

The impact of poor sleep quality is unavoidable and immediate. Taking a power nap from time to time is important. If you find yourself with sleeping difficulties, it is recommended that you take supplements to boost your sleep. Such supplements will help to relieve you of nervousness and anxiety which can hinder you from falling and remaining asleep for long.

10.4 Does Exercise Aid In Hair Loss Prevention?

Eating a healthy diet and exercising can prevent certain type of hair loss that doesn't result from aging. In most cases, this kind of hair loss is caused by stress and it is easily reversible if the right actions are taken on time. However, if you experience hair loss, the first and most important thing to do is to visit a doctor to get some professional advice about the right treatment for you.

Normally, hair follicles undergo through three growth phases. This kind of growth cycle is highly affected by effluviums or hair loss conditions. Another important type of hair loss is telogen effluvium that results when the number of hair follicles on your head changes. Thankfully, it is easy to reverse telogen effluvium as it rarely results in overall balding. Medical professionals and hair follicle experts say that loss of hair can be sustained by shocking the hair follicles and this is where the importance of exercise in hair loss prevention comes in. Alternatively, you can use other strategies to shock the hair follicles such as through hormonal changes, crash diets, surgery and physical trauma.

The two major causes of hair loss have been described to be poor dieting and chronic stress. Based on this, it is clear that you can prevent some forms of hair loss through exercise. In case your loss of hair results from inadequate nutrition or stress, a lifestyle change can help you in dealing with the situation. This involves incorporation of a healthy eating regime and doing some exercises that can reverse hair loss and prevent the hair from being shed off.

However, the bottom line and what you should keep in mind as you exercise is that not all forms of hair loss can be prevented through exercise. As such, if you find your situation not improving after incorporating exercises in your daily life, it is essential that you visit a hair specialist for alternative treatments. You can try your luck with natural treatments or artificial medications and find out what works best for you.

Exercises play a significant role in enhancing adequate circulation of blood and essential nutrients for hair growth to the scalp. The blood carries nutrients that it distributes throughout the body through circulation including the scalp. By increasing blood flow or blood circulation, it is possible to provide your hair with the necessary nutrients required for growth and thus prevent hair loss. Exercises boost flow of blood to the head which prevents hair loss and encourages growth of healthy hair.

Cardiovascular exercises boost the pumping action of the head and sends nutrients and oxygen to the head. Other essential exercises to consider are such as walking, aerobics, running, swimming and yoga.

10.5 How To Eat A Clean Diet

There is no overnight cure for hair loss, but you can encourage healthy hair growth with clean diet. Eating clean is a concept that has been with us for ages now. A cleaner diet is definitely not a fad diet for weight loss. When it comes to eating a clean diet, this requires that you stick to eating foods that are natural and avoid eating processed foods which you buy at the fast food joint. In addition, a clean diet doesn't require that you restrict yourself on what you are eating but it is all about making conscious choices by eating high quality foods. A clean diet as such means eating more natural products while minimizing your intake for additives and chemicals.

While some people are actually able to start eating clean without looking back, most people tend to find it hard trying to adapt to this lifestyle. A good place to start when thinking about eating a clean diet is to start drinking more water. Next, work towards eliminating processed foods and then try to balance your meals as you work towards controlling your portion sizes. Putting more water in your body is of great importance as far as your health wellness is concerned. Unfortunately, most people tend to underestimate the importance of drinking more water. They end up considering drinking of other drinks such as sodas as a substitute for water. Such a baseless myth must be put to an end and you must understand that other liquids are not the same as water.

The next important aspect of eating a clean diet is to work hard towards eliminating processed foods from your daily diet. Food that has gone through more process is very bad for your health. The body has been designed to easily absorb natural products with minimal processing requirements. You can start by eliminating sugar and substituting it with honey as refined sugar is a great threat to your health. Also, practice a healthy eating habit buying fresh fruits and vegetables rather than using frozen food products. Eat fresh meat instead of going for pre- packaged meat. Lean meat contain high amount of proteins and it is good for your health such as turkey breast and chicken.

The other step is to balance your meals properly. The general guidelines require that about 50 percent of your meal should be made of carbohydrates, 15 percent fats and 35 percent proteins. The fact is that your body requires all these nutrients for proper functioning along with water, minerals and vitamins. For the best results, all these nutrients must be provided to the body in the best proportions and if you can manage to maintain that on regular basis, it is possible to see your body performing to its full potential.

In conclusion, don't expect to find a magic diet which can make you get fit and avoid common health problems. Eating a clean diet might not be easy but if you are able to stick by it without worrying about perfection, you are going to do your body a lot of justice including healthy hair growth.

10.6 Benefits of Proteins for Healthy Hair Growth

It is mandatory to include proteins in your regular diet. This is because proteins are the structural components in the body cells and thus play a critical role in ensuring that our system functions properly and as required. On average, an adult is advised to eat between 1.4 and 2.5 ounces of proteins on a daily basis. However, this often varies depending on various factors such as height and weight of the person. For instance, people suffering from diseases and weak immunity are advised to increase their protein intake as the body badly needs it to repair damaged cells as it constructs new ones.

Furthermore, proteins play a vital role in healthy hair development. There is a very close relationship between growth of robust and healthy hair and proteins. It is widely known that almost 80 percent of a person's hair comprises of a protein known as keratin. This protein is made up of polypeptide chains and two amino acids joined together. According to dermatologists and hair specialists, one of the main culprits for hair thinning and hair loss is deficiency of proteins. As such, the hair needs proteins on a daily basis in order to evade this risk that can make you to lose your precious locks. Taking protein rich foods is the best tip that anyone can give you when looking for possible ways to promote faster and healthy hair growth.

As highlighted, human hair strands are majorly composed of proteins and comprise of amino acids. There are twenty amino acids which are involved in the process of synthesizing essential proteins in the body. Our body system produces eleven amino acids while you are supposed to take the remaining amino acids from your diet. As such, if you want to boost your hair growth, your meals should contain these proteins in abundance. Taking these essential amino acids is a must for you to maintain healthy hair growth. As such, if your body lacks the amino acids, it becomes impossible for it to form hair fiber which leads to hair loss and hair thinning and in extreme cases, this can result in baldness.

Protein level in the body can be maintained by taking a diet rich in proteins. You can obtain these proteins from plant sources or non-vegetarian food. Some of animal sources of proteins include meat, fish, eggs, poultry as well as dairy products. Animal sources are regarded as complete proteins as they contain all the nine essential amino acids in sufficient amounts. Some of the plant sources for proteins include grains, legumes, seeds, vegetables and nuts.

Furthermore, you can also take synthetic alternatives as a source of proteins which come in form of supplements. Such protein supplementations not only promote healthy growth of hair but also boost your overall body health as well. However, before you alter your diet in order to incorporate these proteins, always consult your dermatologist first. Also, you should be careful as researchers warn that too high amounts of protein in the diet can be harmful to your health.

10.7 Learn How to Eat Fresh

It is an obvious fact that fresh foods are the best for our bodies. After all, ingredients and chemicals that some of us can't even pronounce are not always appetizing as they claim. Eating fresh foods helps in reawakening your taste buds that might have been lost being eating flavorful and processed foods. Developing good eating habits is essential in determining your general health wellness. Unfortunately, processed foods are widely available today and trying to eat fresh can be a serious challenge for many people. Even though such processed foods also have some nutritional value, it is not as much compared to fresh foods.

Any kind of food included in the diet contributes in some way to the effectiveness of body functioning. It is thus important to consider including fresh foods in your meals as they supply you with natural minerals and vitamins required by the body to function better. You can only realize the numerous benefits of eating fresh food by trying them and ascertaining the kind of impact they have on your healthy. Such a healthier eating lifestyle should include fresh sources of vegetables and fruits, fish, grains and meats. By incorporating this in the diet, you will not just feel a great difference in your body but you will also empower your immune system such that it can fight off diseases.

Fresh foods are known to contain high amounts of vitamins which are supplied directly into the body. Such vitamins are usually destroyed when food is processed and fresh food is always the best. Also, when you buy fruits, vegetables, crisp leaves and firm flesh, it is always important to think of its nutritional value and supply your body with the best foods. Poultry and meat should always smell fresh, have a good texture, maintain color consistency and look bright. Another important food in a diet is fish. When you are buying fish at the grocery, ensure it is fresh and look into its eyes to determine its freshness. A fresh fish will have clear look in the eyes. Addition, all seafood have more nutritional value when taken fresh and should of course be having a good smell.

Consumption of diets rich in sugary and starchy foods not only leads excessive weight gain but also leads to deficiencies that can interfere with healthy development of your hair. In the worst case scenario, such foods contribute to health difficulties and shorten your life span greatly. For that reason, the importance of eating fresh cannot be overstated as it has great benefit on your health. And in any case, you will realize that eating fresh is also cost effective and very beneficial in many other ways.

If you consider the number of times you feel sick after eating processed food, you will realize why fresh foods are the best choice. These foods especially vegetables and fruits strengthen your immune system thus preventing sickness and other common conditions like flu and cold. This way you can grow healthy hair.

10.8 Useful Detox Diet Tips

Detoxification can help in stopping hair loss and promoting hair growth at the same time. Detoxification helps in giving your hair a new start by eliminating harmful chemicals and getting rid of chemicals that inhibit hair growth. This involves making your scalp, oil glands, roots and hair follicles free from elements that hinder hair re-growth. Detox helps on reversing chemical damages caused by use of synthetic hair treatments and products. By removing these toxins, detoxification helps not only in optimizing hair health but also building up your immune system as well as keeping you free from scalp and hair disease causing poisons that interfere with healthy hair growth.

When you start feeling out of sync, sluggish and having some skin problems, pains, aches and hair loss, these are signs that your body needs a detox. Detoxification is a concept that has been practice for many centuries by so many cultures all over the world even the Chinese and ayurvedic medicine systems. To detox the body is all about cleaning, nourishing and resting the body from inside out. By eliminating and removing these toxins and then feeding the body with some healthy nutrients, detox helps in protecting the body from diseases and renewing its ability to support optimum health.

Health experts will tell you that the body has a natural healing system that is enhanced and strengthened through detoxification. In the most basic aspect of it, detoxification means blood cleansing. This is mainly accomplished by removal of blood impurities especially in the liver which processes toxins for elimination. In addition, the body is also able to eliminate the toxins through intestines, kidneys lymph, skin and lungs. However, ingesting impurities tend to compromise this natural process and this can affect all the body cells adversely.

Adopting an effective detox program helps in cleaning the body by resting the organs, stimulating the ability of the liver to eliminate toxins and also promoting elimination of the impurities through the skin, kidneys and the intestines. Detoxification is also very useful in improving blood circulation to the hair follicles and refueling the body through healthy nutrients. What makes detoxification to work effectively is the fact that it addresses the specific requirements of the individual cells. You can detox your body by use of cleansing supplement packages which contain vitamins, fiber, minerals and herbs. Another approach of body detoxification involves developing a routine of taking plenty of water on a daily basis.

You can detox and cleanse the body though lifestyle supplements, diets and supplements. Eating plenty of fiber from brown rice, vegetables and fresh fruits grown organically is an excellent way to detox the body. Other essential foods in this area are such as beets, artichokes, radishes, broccoli, cabbage, chlorella, spirulina and seaweed. Herbs like burdock, milk thistle and dandelion root also help in protecting and cleansing the liver. Vitamin C also helps the body in production of glutathione, a special compound in the liver that flushes away toxins from the body.

The role that water plays when it comes to body detox cannot be assumed and it is essential that you develop a habit of drinking at least 8 glasses of water daily. It is also advisable that you breathe deeply in order to allow better circulation of oxygen in your body system. Emphasizing on your positive emotions also helps in stress transformation. Sweating in the sauna aids the body in elimination of wastes through the process of perspiration. Lastly, any good detox program must also include exercises. Jumping around, walking, running, dancing, biking and yoga are great accesses that also help your body to stay fit. Detoxification has awesome health benefits that you definitely shouldn't miss.

Detoxing helps your hair in very many ways as chemicals are known to cause a lot of damage to hair follicles. However, the health of your hair also depends on your overall health and by removing the toxins and harmful chemicals, your entire body health stays on top gear.

10.9 Vitamins, Minerals and Specials Nutrition for Better Hair Growth

Nutritional food substances have very beneficial effects on growth of health hair and helps in re-establishment of hair on bald sections. According to past studies, there is a clear evident that people with a good nutrition habit have healthier hair. It was revealed that such people's diet is rich in fresh fruits and vegetables and whole beans and grains in addition to consuming less red meats and animal proteins.

Minerals and vitamins have high nutritional value especially when it comes to promoting healthy growth of hair. One of the healthy hair vitamins you should take is Vitamin A which is a very effective antioxidant that boosts the production of sebum on the scalp. You can get this vitamin from fish liver oil, milk, meat, spinach, eggs, cheese, carrots, cabbage, broccoli, peaches and apricots. Vitamin C is yet another very important vitamin for better hair growth and plays a critical role in maintenance of healthy skin and hair. You can obtain Vitamin C from citrus fruits, kiwi, strawberries, pineapple, cantaloupe, green peppers, tomatoes, dark green vegetables and potatoes.

It is also not a secret that Vitamin E enhances circulation of blood in the scalp and can be obtained from wheat germ oil, raw seeds, nuts, soybeans and dried beams. However, research also shows that this vitamin can induce clotting of the blood and can also increase blood pressure. Biotin vitamin aids in production of keratin that prevents hair loss and graying. You can get this vitamin from milk, rice, liver, grains and egg yolks as well as whole grains. Inositol vitamin maintains the healthiness of hair follicles at cellular level and it is recommended that you eat citrus fruits to get this vitamin in sufficient quantities.

Besides vitamins, minerals are also very important for healthy hair growth especially calcium which is obtained from fish, dairy, lentils and tofu. However, avoid excessive intake of calcium as it can inhibit absorption of iron and zinc. Chromium is another important mineral that helps to prevent hypoglycemia and hyperglycemia which are very notorious in accelerating hair loss. Copper is another very essential mineral that contributes greatly in preventing defects in the structure and color of the hair. However, high dosages of copper can lead to development of dry hair while also causing other more serious health problems.

Iodine helps in regulation of thyroid hormones while also preventing loss of hair and dryness. Iodine is found in sufficient quantities in fish, garlic, iodized salt and kelp. Iron is not only useful in preventing anemia but also prevents loss of hair. However, just like calcium, too much iron can result in malfunction of spleen and the liver. Other essential minerals that you should include in your nutrition regime are such as zinc, sulfur, silica, selenium and potassium. Taking such a special nutrition will help to improve your hair and promote your general health wellness as well. However, consistency and patience is important in order to see considerable results.

10.10 Scalp Massage and Cleansing

Massaging and cleansing of the hair are two largely overlooked aspects of proper hair care that are vitally important. They are critical aspects of rejuvenation and maintenance of hair alongside taking a proper diet to promote healthy hair growth and using holistic and organic shampoos. Cleansing helps to eliminate waste materials like uric acid deposits and catarrh crystals that can inhibit proper hair growth. When such impurities build up on the scalp, they can easily lead to hair fall and negatively affect the health of your hair.

Massaging the scalp also stimulates capillaries and enhances circulation of blood to the head thus boosting transportation of nutrients and oxygen. Most importantly, massaging and cleansing stimulates oil and hormone producing glands on the scalp. This helps in keeping the skin pores on the head to remain open all the time for breathing and aids in retention of natural oils. Hair loss can at times be traced back to sebaceous glands which produce natural oil for lubrication of the hair. When these glands are not in balance, what follows is either over production or under production of sebum that affects the natural hair growth process. In either case, this interferes with nourishment of hair roots and weakens the scalp which leads to falling of the hair on its own. When the hair follicles are under nourished, the hair becomes brittle and dry and starting falling out.

At other times, foreign matter obtained from gels, mousses, artificial conditioners and shampoos as well as hair sprays tend to clog the follicles and pores. These chemicals are very dangerous and besides interfering with natural nourishment of hair roots, they seriously disrupt the normal hair growth process. Such chemicals are absorbed in the blood stream as well and circulated to other body parts which can negatively impact on your health wellness. Massaging and cleansing the hair is a great way to stay off such problems. Due to its nourishing effects on the scalp and hair, massaging is like using a dry shampoo and if done appropriately, it can act as a very effective natural conditioner.

While stimulating sebaceous glands, massaging promotes distribution of sebum all over the scalp and hair. This makes the hair more resilient, manageable and stronger. In addition, by ensuring that the hair is coated with sebum, massaging also prevents moisture from evaporating excessively from the scalp thus giving the hair a more natural texture and sheen. Massaging and cleansing should be done at least twice in a day using a natural scalp massager. It is highly advisable that you avoid using artificial or plastic ones as they can be very invasive on the scalp.

When cleansing your hair, use an idea brush depending on the sensitivity and thickness of your hair and scalp. More often than not, using a brush with soft bristle helps in soothing your head and enlivening its effect on the scalp. For ultimate rejuvenation and maintenance of your hair, it is essential to have a regular schedule for scalp massage and cleansing for best results.

11. Medicated Treatments for Hair Loss

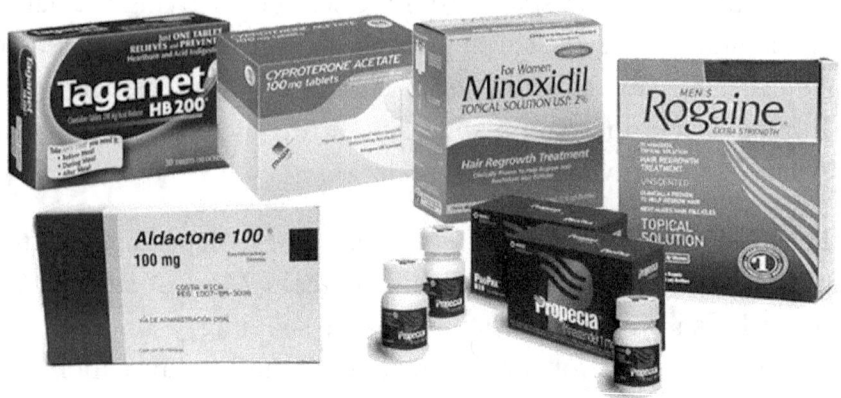

11.1 Minoxidil Topical Treatment

Minoxidil topical treatment is used to slow balding and stimulate growth of hair. This treatment is most effective when used by people aged below 40 years with a recent hair loss. Doctors say that Minoxidil doesn't have any notable effects on a receding hairline. Additionally, this treatment is not a cure for baldness. Once the usage of the drug has been stopped, most of the new hair gets lost so it is important that you continue using it once you have started. Basically, Minoxidil topical treatment is available in liquid for and it is applied orally on the scalp. For best results, it should be applied twice in a day by the patient.

When using Minoxidil, it is essential that all the directions of usage are followed carefully as prescribed on the label. Using less or more treatment than advised by the doctor is highly discouraged.

Exceeding the doctor's recommended dosage doesn't produce faster or greater hair growth not to forget that it can cause serious side effects. Besides, the treatment must be used for a period not less than four months and for about 1 year before any meaningful effects can be seen. Upon purchasing Minoxidil topical treatment, you will be provided with 3 special applicators.

For large scalp sections, use the metered spray applicator and the rub on applicator and extended spray applicator can be used for treating small scalp areas. Minoxidil should only be applied to the scalp and dry hair. As such, avoid using the treatment on your other body areas and most importantly, keep the drug away from sensitive skin and eyes. In case it gets into contact with such areas accidentally, wash the area with a lot of cool water and consult your doctor if possible. Also, Minoxidil topical treatment shouldn't be applied on irritated or sunburned scalp as it can have devastating results.

Minoxidil has been observed to have some side effects and you should visit your doctor in case the symptoms become severe and fail to go away. Some of the common side effects include scalp itching, scaling, dryness, burning sensation, irritation or flaking. Other more serious side effects include weight gain, breathing difficulties, swelling of face, hands, stomach and ankles, rapid heartbeat, lightheadedness and chest pain.

Minoxidil topical treatment is commercially sold under the brand name of Rogaine and it is one of the most effective treatments as far as promoting hair growth is concerned. However, always remember that Rogaine is only intended for external use and strictly not internal. As such, do not swallow Minoxidil and do not apply bandages, dressings, lotions, cosmetics and other alternative skin medications on treated areas. If you are using other medications for hair growth besides Minoxidil topical treatment, it is essential that you maintain a written wrist showcasing all your nonprescription and prescription medicines you are using. This also includes other hair growth dietary supplements, minerals and vitamins that you could be using. You should consult your doctor in case you notice any undesirable side effects.

11.2 Aldactone/Spironolactone Treatment

While Aldactone/spironolactone can help people especially women experiencing hair loss problems as a result of hormonal imbalance, this treatment is not meant for everyone. As such, before you consider buying this drug, this e-book will help you know whether you are an ideal candidate for this treatment or not.

Some women tend to lose their hair due to overproduction of the male hormones in their bodies. If you are a victim of this, Aldactone is useful drug to consider using. Female pattern hair loss can result from many problems. This condition leads to gradual thinning of the hair over time and in the long run, it results in bare or thin patches on the top of head or at the front of scalp. Such kind of hair loss is also known as the androgenetic hair loss and worsens after menopause for most women and is normally hereditary.

This kind of hair loss is normally caused by presence of higher than normal androgen levels in the body. This hormone is only available in very small quantities in women while men produce it in large quantities. Also, some women can also develop increased sensitivity to male hormones like testosterone and this can cause hair loss. For instance, women suffering from PCOS or polycystic ovary syndrome tend to produce androgens in more quantities. This can result in growth of hair on facial areas while leading to loss of hair on the head alongside other health problems like metabolic complications and infertility.

This is where Aldactone/spironolactone comes in and helps in restoration of hormonal balance while treating female pattern hair loss among women. However, Aldactone is not specifically approved for use as a hair loss treatment. As such, even if the doctor recommends it to you, always remember that it is an off label treatment but can still help. Aldactone is basically effective potassium sparing diuretic meaning that it is capable of getting rid of excess body fluids just like other water pills/diuretics do. However, it doesn't make its users lose a lot of potassium in the process like other diuretics do. Primarily, the drug is used for treating high blood pressure, potassium deficiency and swelling.

However, based on the fact that Aldactone/spironolactone works as an effective anti- androgen, this drug acts as a treatment for women suffering from hair loss due to increased androgen levels. The effect of this drug is that it slows down the production of androgens in the ovaries and adrenal glands while also inhibiting the action of produced androgens. Mostly, Aldactone/ spironolactone accomplishes this by combating dihydrotesterone -this refers to the specific form of testosterone which is responsible for causing hair loss- and prevents it from binding to the androgenetic receptor which could affect hair follicles.

Keep in mind that Aldactone/spironolactone is not going to help you in growing new hair. However, it helps thinning hair to become fuller and thicker which makes it one of the most effective treatments for hair loss and hair thinning.

11.3 Tagamet/Cimetidine Treatment

Cimetidine is characterized as an antagonist for histamine H2. It is commonly referred to as Tagamet or a histamine blocker. Primarily, this oral medication aids in reduction of stomach acids and this helps in treating both gastric ulcers and duodenal. In addition, it is a proven fact that Cimetidine is also very beneficial when sued by sufferers of acid indigestion and heartburn. However, when used in higher doses, Cimetidine has been found to affect levels of the male sex hormones/ androgens in the body. As such, this encourages growth of hair among women experiencing androgenetic alopecia or female pattern baldness.

Even though female pattern baldness is caused by a wide range of factors, hair specialists note that DHT or dihydrotestosterone is the most common cause of this condition in most cases. Exposing testosterone to an enzyme called type II 5 alpha reductase converts this hormone to DHT. DHT then binds itself to hair follicles which are very sensitive to the hormone and triggers miniaturization and can result in subsequent loss of hair. When this happens, this is where Cimetidine comes in. According to hair loss experts, Cimetidine majorly acts as a highly effective antiandrogenetic where by it inhibits biological effects of the male sex hormones in the body. Using Tagamet/Cimetidine on a daily basis aids in lowering the levels of testosterone in the woman's body and thus leads to reduced DHT levels. When the scalp has less DHT, this leads to a reduction in progression of loss of hair and also promotes hair re-growth. In addition, cimetidine also prevents DHT from being attached on hair follicles which can trigger loss of hair due to shrinkage.

For best results, Cimetidine must be used taken in an appropriate dosage as recommended by the doctor. However, when being used to treat loss of hair among women, Cimetidine should be taken in relatively higher quantities unlike when being used for treatment of gastrointestinal issues. As such, this over the counter medication shouldn't be taken to promote hair growth without doctor's advice as this would mean use of an overdose. A dermatologist can prescribe the right dosage to you and help avoid unwanted side effects. Also, the prescription tends to vary from one woman to another but just like any other medication, you must follow orders given by the doctor.

Cimetidine might not be the ultimate solution and at times, it might fail to produce desired results. At other times, the doctor might determine that this treatment is not appropriate for you and you should consider using other effective medications that promote hair growth. Androgenetic alopecia can be treated successfully by a range of other treatments such as Minoxidil, oral contraceptives, spironolactone, ketoconazole and hormone replacement therapy among other treatments that are equally promising in dealing with hair loss as highlighted in this e-book. However, men must never use Cimetidine to promote re-growth of hair. Use of higher dosages can lead to adverse effects in men and can cause disastrous side effects including feminization.

11.4 Cyproterone Acetate Treatment

Products made using Cyproterone acetate offer an alternative treatment for women hair loss and include brand names such as Androcur, Dianette, Cyprone, Andro- Diane, Diane 35, Diane 50 and Cyprostate. These are basically products which contain Cyproterone acetate as the main/ active ingredient in them. This hair loss medication is basically based on hormone referred to as antiandrogen which lowers down testosterone levels in the body. However, even though there is evidence that Cyproterone acetate can actually treat hair loss and promote hair growth, the medication is not approved.

In other platforms, Cyproterone acetate is used for controlling effects of testosterone hormone. Among men, the medication is used for treating hyper sexuality while also helping in management of overactive sex drive. Also, doctors recommend the use of this medication in managing symptoms of prostate cancer. In women, Cyproterone acetate is given as a prescription to deal with excess growth of hair on the body or loss of hair on the scalp due to increased levels of the male hormones. The medication is combined with another hormone known as the ethinyl estradiol to for a birth control pill that is given as a prescription to women. Such contraceptives are sold under various brand names such as Dianette, Diane 50 or Diane 35.

Alongside its derivatives, Cyproterone acetate is very effective in treatment of female pattern hair loss. It accomplishes this by blocking the reaction of the male hormone on the hair follicles which can lead to hair falling off. To be more precise, Cyproterone acetate functions by minimizing the effects of testosterone on the hair follicles. This way, it helps to prevent loss of hair triggered by imbalance of testosterone hormone in women. When present in a woman body, these male hormones lead to miniaturization of hair follicles and causes hair to fall off from the scalp. By blocking this action, the hair does not get miniaturized and increases the density and volume of hair in its place.

Unfortunately, despite this revelation of Cyproterone acetate being known, this medication is not available as a prescription drug for treating hair loss. However, you can still use one of its many varieties to combat the hair loss problem. Cyproterone acetate was initially introduced on the market in the 1970's. However, despite its effectiveness in controlling reproduction, hair loss and acne, this medication is not without its share of controversy. For instance, women who have been using Cyproterone acetate of late have reported risk of blood clotting especially when taken as a contraceptive.

Using Cyproterone acetate without a doctor's advice is highly discouraged. It has a potential of causing other risks such as damaging the liver, mood changes/ depression and can also cause erectile dysfunction and enlarged breasts among men. Even though Cyproterone acetate actually treats loss of hair, it is unlikely that the product will soon be available as a hair loss prescription due to the high cost of getting the drug approved by the Food and Drug Administration Board.

11.5 Estrogen/Progesterone Treatment

There is quite a wide range of reasons and factors responsible for hair loss including a dramatic or sudden change in hormonal levels in the body. The ovaries produce these hormones and are responsible for carrying out vital functions in the body ranging from providing you with assistance during pregnancy period and regulating other hormones in the body. If you are worried that you are suffering from a hormonal imbalance that could result in loss of hair, you should see your doctor as soon as possible. There are so many causes of hair loss and it is necessary that you get the right treatment for your specific condition.

Estrogen and progesterone are at times used during the process of hormonal therapy and helps women in relieving menopause symptoms. In absence of both estrogen and progesterone hormones, a woman is exposed to the risk of suffering from osteoporosis, hot flashes, dry skin, vaginal dryness, bladder dryness, hair loss and sleeplessness. In fact, doctors are categorical on the fact that presence of both estrogen and progesterone hormone in low levels can easily result in female pattern baldness and hair loss.

There are many times when a woman can experience fluctuation of hormones in her body including during menopause, pregnancy and puberty periods. However, loss of hair among women is most common during menopause and after pregnancy as this is the period when estrogen and progesterone hormones decrease dramatically. According to hair specialists, it is most likely that loss of hair occurs 3 months after post partum. During this time, a woman is more prone to hair loss as there is a significant drop in hormonal levels after giving birth. During the entire pregnancy period, the hormones continue climb and once the baby is born, they drop drastically. These two hormones also suffer a similar fate during menopause and this is the cause of the numerous side effects experienced by women during menopause.

If you are experiencing loss of hair due to low levels of estrogen and progesterone especially after giving birth, this condition should only occur for a period of between 6 and 12 months and no further, depending upon the levels of the hormones in your body. As such, this kind of hair loss is just temporary and you don't even need to use any kind of treatment. However, for women in menopause period, it is worthwhile to consider hormonal therapy as a solution to the problem. Hormonal therapy helps in restoring the level of estrogen and progesterone in the body which helps to decelerate hair loss.

Even though going for a hormonal therapy is recommended, you should also keep in mind the fact that loss of hair can also be caused by other medical conditions, genetics and certain medications. As such, do not just assume that estrogen and progesterone hormones are to blame for your loss without seeing a physician. Fluctuation of estrogen and progesterone especially due discontinued use of birth control can cause hormonal fluctuation that can then trigger hair loss problems.

11.6 Oral Contraceptives

Oral contraceptives have been identified as a cause of hair loss in some women. However, for other women especially those with androgenetic alopecia, oral contraceptives are an effective treatment for hair loss. Men are not the only species that find hair on the comb when brushing or combing their hair and also find bald patches and thinning areas on their scalps. Just like men, women also experience loss of hair and struggle a lot trying to find a reliable treatment for restoring their thick, full hair back.

A condition known as female pattern baldness or androgenetic alopecia is a very common cause of hair loss in women. However, women have several alternatives for treating their hair loss issues including Rogaine or Minoxidil. Recently, a combination of oral contraceptives with another medication has become one of the most popular treatments prescribed for women suffering from androgenetic alopecia. The working of oral contraceptives in curing women hair loss goes back to the issue of hormones. Generally, hormones affect nearly all the processes in the body like hair growth.

Birth control pills or oral contraceptives usually contain hormones which could be either progestin and estrogen or just progestin alone.

These pills prevent the user from getting pregnant by preventing the monthly process of egg release or ovulation. However, these birth control pills can also lower androgen levels, which are male hormones that are available in small levels in women and are largely related to loss of hair. When androgen hormones are available in unusually high levels in women body, they can lead to androgenetic alopecia. Oral contraceptives are normally combined with another treatment, spironolactone/ Aldactone when being used to combat hair loss.

Primarily, spironolactone is a medication for treating high blood pressure. However, studies have shown that it inhibits production of androgen and it thus an effective medication for controlling hair loss. However, just like other medications, oral contraceptives have their benefits and drawbacks when used to treat loss of hair. On their positive aspect, these birth control pills are able to prevent women from getting unwanted pregnancy and can also prevent androgenetic hair loss effectively. However, use of oral contraceptives also comes with a range of side effects, some of which can be disastrous. For starters, these contraceptives increase the risk of heart attack, stroke and blood clots. Other undesirable side effects include increased risk of breast cancer, sore breasts, acne and nausea.

Oral contraceptives are not completely safe for all women and in fact, women aged over 35 years and are smokers can have serious effects by using them like development of blood clots and are not advised to use birth control pills to treat hair loss. Also, not all oral contraceptives are effective in treating loss of hair and some of them can actually make the problem worse or even trigger hair loss. You should only use birth control pills that have a low index of androgen such as Desogen, Ortho-Cyclen, Ortho-Cept and Micronor while avoiding other pills such as Loestrin and Ovral.

11.7 Nizoral Treatment for Female Hair Loss

For the past couple of years, Nizoral hair loss treatment has been debated widely. Marketed as an effective treatment for dandruffs, hair specialists have also found interesting side effects on the relationship between Nizoral and hair loss. Generally, Nizoral contains about 2 percent of Ketoconazole. This medication is primarily used for treating fungal infections. Nizoral hair loss treatment shampoos should be applied on the scalp at least twice in a week and the shampoo should be left on the scalp for about 5 min before rinsing and it will work magic.

The effectiveness of Nizoral as a useful treatment for loss of hair in women is highly attributed to anti-androgenic effects of Ketoconazole. This medication inhibits testosterone production in men and women. As such, if your loss of hair has been triggered by use of testosterone solutions excessively, Nizoral hair loss effective can be very effective on your hair. Men and women experiencing androgenetic alopecia should definitely consider using Nizoral shampoos to treat their hair loss problems. Perhaps the best thing about Nizoral treatment for hair loss is that there are no any side effects that have been reported. And trying the treatment is also pretty easy. You can simply buy the 2% Nizoral version at an online drugstore without any prescription.

Past studies done about the effectiveness of using Nizoral to treat hair loss are very interesting. For instance, a study completed in 1998 concluded that the desirable effects of using Nizoral containing 2 percent Ketoconazole was the same as using the well known topical Minoxidil. However, this study was only carried out in men and there is absolutely no guarantee of similar results among women. And even so, FDA wasn't convinced enough by these results to endorse Nizoral as a hair loss treatment. Later studies carried out with mice revealed that Ketoconazole which is present in Nizoral aids in stimulating growth of hair.

The researchers speculated that Nizoral functions by impacting on the hormone levels and immune system. In addition, the researchers also noted that it helps in unclogging of hair follicles for the oily deposit known as sebum which inhibits growth of hair. Another side benefit of Nizoral as the researchers found out is that it made hair to appear fuller. Another little known fact about Nizoral is that this treatment is extremely effective when used to treat some of baldness as well. This is thanks to the presence of Ketoconazole that fights baldness aggressively and promotes restoration of hair.

Without any doubts, the relatively low price of Nizoral treatment is a major benefit for users of this product. Actually, the reason why this product is sold at such a low price is that most people still believe that it is just a shampoo for dandruffs and even its manufacturers are yet to market it based on its effectiveness in offering protection against loss of hair. However, always keep in mind that Nizoral slows or stops loss of hair and does not necessarily promote hair re-growth.

11.8 Propecia Vs Proscar Treatment for Male Pattern Hair Loss

Propecia is generally an androgen hormone inhibitor which is marketed for use by men experiencing male pattern baldness. This drug acts on skin receptors on the scalp. Even though Propecia doesn't necessarily promote re-growth of lost hair, it has been found to be very effective in arresting hair loss at early stages for most of its users. For men who have been taking Propecia since their childhood, they can acknowledge that it is one of the most remarkable medications on the market today. Numerous reviews have given this drug thumbs up as it works quite marvelous in preventing a receding hair line. However, it shouldn't be used by pregnant females is it can lead to birth defects. However, as far as men are concerned, Propecia doesn't have any reported side effects.

The same company behind Propecia is also the one that markets another men only drug known as Proscar. At the most basic of it, Proscar is a drug that inhibits production of androgen hormone. Also, men use this drug for treating swelling of their prostate which is a condition referred to as benign prostatic hyperplasia. Proscar should be taken in a dosage of 5 milligrams per day and it can help in dealing with a swelling prostate gland and thus helps in relieving several urinary tract conditions linked to the disease.

The little secret about Propecia and Proscar that most people don't know is that clinical trial have revealed that both of these drugs contain the same active ingredient. This should hint to you why the two are effective in dealing with male pattern hair loss despite being marketed for different conditions. If you go to a hair loss specialist and prescribe to you Propecia, you will be given finasteride which contains Propecia, the active ingredient that inhibits androgen hormone. If you visit a doctor seeking treatment for your prostate cancer/ enlarged prostate, chances are high that you will be prescribed Proscar. You will then have to buy finasteride for the active ingredient.

As such, this drug company sells exactly the same active ingredient but for two different purposes. This marvelous active ingredient thus has the capability of treating prostate cancer and also treating male pattern hair loss. Most men who have been using finasteride for baldness have acknowledged great satisfaction on the effectiveness of the drug in dealing with their hair loss condition. In short, both Propecia and Proscar is one and the same drug even though the tablets come in different shapes and color.

The bottom line is that both Proscar and Propecia are effective and safe drugs for their specific purposes. If you are suffering from male pattern hair loss, you can definitely find relief in Propecia and get to see your conditions treated. The good attributes about the drug is that besides being cheap and affordable, it is very safe and effective in treating male pattern hair loss. As such, you can forget about suffering from any undesirable side effects out of its use.

11.9 Cyproterone Acetate with Ethinylestradiol

Manufactured by Bayer, Cyproterone acetate with ethinylestradiol is marketed under the brand name of Dianette and primarily used to treat severe hirsutism and acne in women. This hormone contraceptive pill for women is also used for treating abnormal hair growth among women. Cyproterone acetate is a medication referred to as an anti androgen. As you already know, androgens are the male hormones which are produced by both men and women. The hormones are responsible for promoting skin growth including hair growing on the skin.

If your body produces androgen in high quantities or your skin is highly sensitive to androgen effects, the sebaceous glands tend to produce a lot of sebum. As a result, hair follicles on your scalp become blocked and could result in inflammation, acne spots or infection. Also, blocking of hair follicles inhibits growth of hair and can cause hair loss and hair thinning on your scalp. Also, presence of androgen hormone in a woman's body causes excessive hair growth especially on the face as well as in other body parts apart from head. The excessive growth of facial hair in women is referred to as hirsutism condition.

Cyproterone acetate with ethinylestradiol helps in preventing the actions of androgens in a woman body. It functions by blocking body receptors where androgens mostly work on. As such, even if androgens are present in high levels, they are not able to affect you skin, cause acne of lead to excessive hair growth on the face or diminished hair growth on the scalp. Additionally, Cyproterone acetate with ethinylestradiol also lowers the production of the male hormones by woman ovaries and as such, there is less circulation of male hormones in the body.

After using this treatment, you will notice that your skin starts to become less greasy within the first few weeks of treatment. However, it will take you a couple of months before you can start witnessing an improvement in your excessive hair growth or acne condition. In addition, Cyproterone acetate with ethinylestradiol is also used as a combined oral contraceptive pill and it is very effective. Cyproterone acetate is basically derived from progestogen while ethinylestradiol ingredient is actually a synthetic form of oestrogen hormone that occurs naturally. This medication prevents eggs in the ovaries from ripening and being released which could result in pregnancy.

Cyproterone acetate with ethinylestradiol is mostly used by women suffering from severe acne and unable to respond to oral antibiotics. Production of the male sex hormones in women can result in hirsutism or abnormal growth of hair on the body but this condition can also be arrested with the medication. Use of this medication also comes with a share of side effects as well. For instance, first time users of Cyproterone acetate with ethinylestradiol can experience irregularities in their menstrual cycle like missed periods, breakthrough bleeding and spotting. However, researchers have found that women using the medication have reduced risks of suffering from breast cancer which is a bonus benefit of using Cyproterone acetate with ethinylestradiol.

12. Natural Remedies for Hair Loss

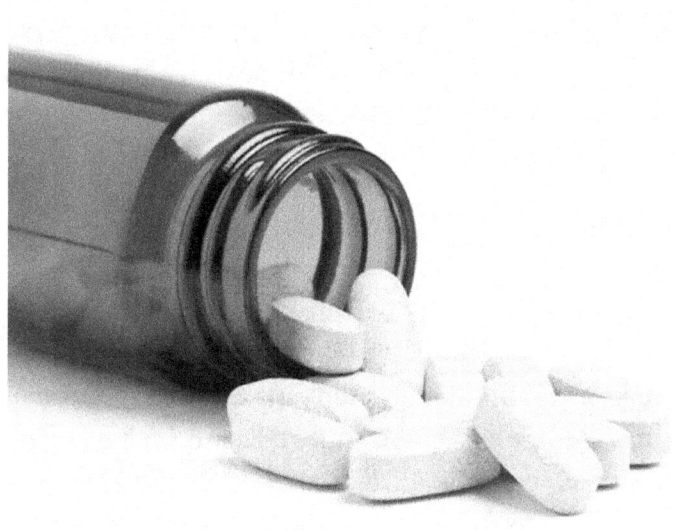

12.1 Multivitamin Supplements for Hair Growth

When dietary problems set in resulting from health issues and poor nutritional habits, getting the proper minerals and vitamins proves to be quite a challenge. Mineral and vitamin deficiency can cause serious loss of hair but consuming a healthy and balanced diet can help to reverse this. Since it might be difficult to get the needed vitamins in your diet, you can use certain vitamin supplements purchased over the counter and could be of significant help to you.

One of the best multivitamin supplements available on the market is vitamin B7 or Biotin. By using this multivitamin regularly, it makes your nails and hair more vibrant and stronger. Other B vitamins are also very important in promoting hair growth such as B6 which binds to testosterone receptors and prevents them from making the hair follicles diminished. Given the large number of multivitamin supplements being marketed today and claiming to promote hair growth, you might tend to think that you will never come across a thinning head or receding hairline anywhere on the streets. However, this is unfortunately not the case.

As far as multivitamin supplements for hair growth are concerned, if you are not seriously experiencing a vitamin deficient, there is no prove that use of these supplements can change your thinning hair in anyway. However, if you seriously have a vitamin deficient, you should consider taking multivitamin supplements. It is important that you identify the specific vitamin/s you are lacking. Thankfully, most hair growth supplements contain a kind of B vitamin known as biotin. Blood tests will help show if you have a deficiency of vitamin D, iron or zinc, all which affect hair growth and other fundamental functions of your body related to your general health wellness. Restoring these nutrients to their normal range will definitely help in boosting your hair density.

Other multivitamin supplements that claim to be the best hair growing products normally include vitamin C, Vitamin A, Vitamin E, amino acids and omega 3 fatty acids. All these are key ingredients in most multivitamin supplements including the prenatal vitamins which can remarkably promote your hair growth. Remember that your hair grows naturally at roughly half an inch every month and it might be difficult to accelerate its growth faster than this even when using multivitamin supplements. As such, even as you use faster hair growth supplements, remember to take basic care of your hair by avoiding heat and chemicals as well as trimming split eats.

While using multivitamin supplements, you should be patient and don't expect any overnight changes. If you are considering using a vitamin/mineral supplement to minimize your hair loss, always consult your doctor/ hair specialist first. Also, only get your multivitamin supplements from trusted sources like a general nutrition center, grocery store or pharmacy. Generally, multivitamin supplements helps in making your scalp and hair stronger and healthier. They help in making your hair more beautiful by supplying your hair follicles with essential nutrients needed for fast and health hair growth.

12.2 Herbal Remedies

Every day, your head loses between 50 and 100 hair strands and dermatologists say this is perfectly normal. However, when the loss exceeds the figure, you start noticing bald patches or hair thinning. Even though there are so many treatments for hair loss on the market today, going herbal might prove to be a lasting solution for your loss. There is quite a wide range of herbal remedies that have been proved to facilitate hair re-growth and are worth a try.

The first herbal remedy is the onion and garlic. These two contains the element of sulphur which specialists say that it increases production of collagen that helps to promote hair growth. Since ancient times, onion and garlic have been used to boost hair re-growth. You just need to chop your onion into small pieces and then squeeze out the juice. Apply it to your scalp gently and rinse it after 15 minutes.

Coconut oil is another herbal remedy that delivers great results as it contains vast ingredients which condition the hair naturally and promote hair growth. The coconut milk contains essential fats, proteins and minerals like iron and potassium. By using coconut milk regularly, this can cause hair breakage in addition to making hair strands strong right all the way from the roots to the shaft and tip. Henna is an herbal remedy that has been in use in Asian countries for hair conditioning and coloring. Henna plays a major role in hair strengthening and works even much better when mixed with mustard oil.

The secret to having a thick hair mane as observed in people who live in Kerala in India is using a combination of hibiscus and coconut oil. Hibiscus is well known for its rejuvenating properties and nourishes hair while also preventing premature graying of hair. In addition, regular use of hibiscus not only prevents loss of hair but it is also a great cure for dandruffs. Amla herbal remedy comes packed with essential antioxidants and vitamin C that acts as a perfect remedy for many hair loss woes. In addition to applying amla on your scalp, it can also be consumed regularly as vitamin C is a vital requirement for your overall health wellness.

More often than not, hair loss and hair thinning result from consumption of a poor diet or not taking good care of your hair. As such, it is essential you ensure that you eat a balanced and healthy diet in order to supply your hair will essential nutrients. Also, you should avoid using harsh chemicals and shampoos as they can lead to hair breakage. Wherever possible, always consider substituting mild herbal shampoos with treatments containing synthetic compounds. By massaging your hair regularly with these herbal oils, you will start noticing great results. By adopting an appropriate hair care regimen while using some of these herbal remedies regularly, you can expect to see a significant improvement in the condition of your hair and forget about hair loss.

12.3 Coconut Oil Treatment

While people greatly desire to become hairy- headed, not so many of them remember how some simple natural things can make a difference in their hair condition. Instead of purchasing dangerous and expensive hair care treatments that contain harsh chemicals, coconut oil has vast benefits that can be a great blessing for your hair. Coconut oil is highly effective for all types of hair. In fact, it is a natural hair conditioner that most people are yet to discover. Coconut oil is found as an ingredient in most hair care products as it helps in promoting re-growth of damaged hair.

Coconut oil is derived from a mature fruit of a coconut tree. The white and thick semi solid oil needs to be warmed first before being used for hair. Generally, coconut oil can be used both internally and externally for ideal skin, hair growth and other benefits. Also, pure, virgin and unrefined coconut oil is a perfect choice for promoting health wellness. For starters, coconut oil gets deep into the hair follicles and nourishes the hair thus promoting its growth. In addition, the oil also promotes the health wellness of your scalp by fighting against various problems like dandruffs, lice and bites that could interfere with healthy hair growth.

For dry hair, coconut oil acts as a moisturizer and also adds shininess, softness and luster to the hair. When used regularly, it also helps in preventing split ends and hair breakage which greatly contribute to increased length of the hair and slows down loss of hair from the scalp. For best results, coconut oil should be applied gently over the hair and scalp. After applying, try to comb your hair through and ensure that you reach each and every strand. In additional, specialists in herbal treatments recommend that you warm the oil first before applying it and then massage the scalp. Leave the coconut oil on the scalp overnight and use a shampoo to wash it in the morning.

Since a hair strand has a tube like structure and it is hollow from inside, the coconut oil penetrates completely into this space. As such, your hair shafts become filled up and acquire more body. In the long run, the hair tends to look fuller and denser and acts as a perfect solution for hair thinning. Hair becomes damaged by shrinking and swelling of fibers due to retention and absorption of water. Coconut oil can help in preventing such kind of hygral fatigue and shields the hair from any possible damages.

Another interesting fact about hair is that it is composed of total protein. As such, loss of proteins from the hair resulting in unhealthy and weak hair but coconut oil can help in reducing such kind of protein loss that can cause hair damage. Researchers have also discovered that coconut oil contains antibacterial properties which protects the scalp and hair from viral/ protozoan/bacteria infections. More so, use of coconut oil helps in preventing graying of hair as well.

12.4 Saw Palmetto

Saw palmetto grows mostly in North America. This dwarf palm plant contains active ingredients that are found in the brown black berries of the plant. For years now, native North Americans have sued saw palmetto for treating breast disorders among women and urinary conditions among men. The plant has also become a popular herbal remedy for loss of hair even though it is yet to be approved by FDA. Its effectiveness in treating loss of hair is based on its similarities with finasteride, a treatment used for enlarged prostates in men. Proscar is used for treating an enlarged prostate which Propecia is used for treating hair loss.

Over the years, saw palmetto has become a popular herbal remedy used for treating a kind of baldness and hair loss known as androgenic alopecia or female and male pattern baldness. It is the kind of hair loss that manifests itself through loss of hair around the temples or top of head. Even though there is no much information on exactly how saw palmetto works, it is believed that ingredients present in saw palmetto works by blocking an enzyme known as 5-alpha reductase from permitting testosterone hormone from being converted to dihydrotestosterone hormone. This hormone is considered to contribute greatly to progression of benign prostatic hyperplasia and androgenic alopecia.

There is also some evidence that suggests that saw palmetto affect sex hormone levels in the body like estrogen and testosterone in other ways. While lab studies show that saw palmetto is an effective remedy for baldness and hair loss, research is underway to determine whether this herb can actually promote growth of hair or stop baldness or loss of hair from progressing. However, just like other herbal remedies and supplements available out there, saw palmetto has its share of side effects as well. The common ones are constipation, mild stomach pain, nausea, diarrhea, bad breath and vomiting. Other people have complained of changes in their sexual desire, breast enlargement or tenderness and erectile dysfunction.

Saw palmetto has been sufficiently tested and found to be an effective treatment for the common benign prostatic hypertrophy. Evidence showing its effectiveness in treating prostate also exists and most doctors have given saw palmetto top rating for dealing with prostate issues. As such, there is strong scientific evidence that saw palmetto supplements can treat hair loss and enlarged breasts.

However, the assumption that most physicians make is that if saw palmetto can effectively treat prostate, it should also well in treating hair loss. However, the use of saw palmetto in treating hair loss is yet to be proved conclusively.

Considering that saw palmetto is not an approved treatment for hair loss, doctors try to give some conjecture estimates as to the proper dosage that should be taken. However, most doctors agree that the average dosage of saw palmetto you should take per day is 320 mg. the bottom line is that saw palmetto is a great natural supplement worthy taking and can be a great solution for your hair loss woes.

12.5 Aloe Treatment

The amazing benefits of using aloe for hair are attributed to the more than 75 known nutrients existing in this herbal remedy. However, other hypothesizers say that aloe barbadensis or aloe Vera contains more than a hundred traceable nutrients. You shouldn't be surprised to know that most organic hair color systems take advantage of aloe Vera as a key ingredient in most of the products retailed on the market today. To start with, aloe works awesomely by promoting hair growth and researchers say that use of aloe for hair growth was started way back by ancient Egyptians.

Aloe is known to contain specific enzymes which promote growth of healthy hair directly. The proteolitic enzymes eradicate the dead skin cells found on the scalp which end up clogging hair follicles and inhibiting its growth. Various conditions such as seborrhea contribute to accumulation of scalp sebum which can trigger partial baldness. The keratolic action of aloe breaks down dead scalp cells and sebum thus promoting further growth of hair. In addition, aloe is known to contain string anti- pruritic properties. These properties aid in alleviation of dryness of the hair and itching of the scalp. Pruritus ailments range from scalp issues to vexing skin and eczema and psoriasis.

This auto immune ailment results after skin cells are produced in excess but aloe can eliminate this condition completely. Besides, aloe reduces itching, scaling, inflammation and redness of the scalp psoriasis and this benefits hair growth directly. Aloe is also reported to harbor key anti- inflammatory properties that reduce inflammation and redness both externally and internally. In fact, it is an undeniable fact that aloe has been used since historical times to treat external wounds and burns as well as an antiseptic that reduces swelling while reducing chances of bacterial infections at the same time

Aloe is also capable of reducing dandruffs thanks to its enzymatic breakdown powers. Dandruffs are caused by a wide range of underlying causes and most doctors attribute the condition majorly to presence of malassezia, a fungus that eats fat and lives on the scalp. Thankfully, aloe boasts of having strong anti fungal properties and thus guarantees and dandruff free scalp. This fungus can only thrive in acidic environment and since aloe has alkalizing properties, it is able to counter such a fungal environment successfully and disallows further buildup and growth of dandruffs.

Aloe also comes with conditioning benefits on the hair. Besides soothing and eliminating any scalp and skin problems, the conditioning properties of aloe are excitingly overwhelming. Aloe leaves produce a gel like substance which has the same chemical composition as keratin, a natural protein found in hair cells. The similarity in structure means that aloe is able to penetrate easily along the hair shaft. In fact, this is the reason why most organic color systems utilize aloe during production of ammonia free hair color.

Aloe also contains over 20 amino acids that acts as building blocks of scalp and hair and adds to the luster and strength of the hair.

12.6 Arnica

A number of celebrities have of late confirmed that they have been using arnica oil for various reasons ranging from maintaining their hair to treating old injuries, child birth scars and for many other reasons. For many centuries now, people have been using arnica as a premier herbal remedy for soothing aching muscles. Another variant of this species as been used by people as healing oil for loss of hair and in tinctures for relaxing stiff muscles and in treatment of wounds.

When using arnica as a relief for hair loss, it is good to note that it should only be used externally as it can be toxic when used internally. Derived from a mountain yellow daisy which mostly grows in Europe, arnica is majorly used for treating bruises. However, arnica oil can also be used to massage the scalp as it reputedly promotes hair growth by stimulating the circulation of blood on the scalp. In addition, arnica oil also stimulates the activity of white blood cells and is thus able to promote healing of scalp infections and also reduces inflammation. As aforementioned here above, arnica shouldn't be taken orally as it can cause toxicity and irritation in the kidneys and gastrointestinal system.

Available in topical gels, pellets as well as massage oil and even in creams, arnica is also used to relieve bleeding and swelling that could result from bruises and blows in the head. When you are involved in a traumatic event, there is a high likelihood that some of your hair might be lost in the process. To prevent this, you should apply and sooth the area with arnica which decreases inflammation while also accelerating recovery. In addition, arnica oil also works great in prevention of cramps.

Today, arnica is among the most useful homeopathic remedies available on the market. In a recent study, it was revealed that the herb actually contains dihydrohelenalin and helenalin which produce effective analgesic and anti inflammatory properties. When applied externally on the scalp, arnica is completely safe oil. Today, there are numerous prepared ointments and salves on the market sold in healthy food stores. Arnica is herb that you can use without wondering whether it is obtained from dried or fresh plant and thus makes it a top favorite among herbalists and clients.

The action of arnica on blood vessels helps in healing and causes re-absorption of blood as a way of preventing bruising and minimizing inflammation. Studies have also shown that arnica oil assists in heart regulation after injury which stops both external and internal hemorrhage. If a hemorrhage occurs on the scalp, this can lead to a serious loss of hair on the affected part of the scalp. As such, the essential and beneficial effects of using arnica oil are very transparent especially due to the incredible healing properties. If you have a bump or bruise on your head, you can support the healing of your skin by using arnica and preventing many hair problems that could arise.

12.7 Jojoba Oil

Of late, jojoba oil has emerged as a mystical relief for fighting hair loss and hair thinning. Even though this oil is not a perfect treatment for hair loss problems, there is no doubt that jojoba oil is an excellent treatment for a coarse and dry hair. In addition, it also comes with natural hair conditioning properties and act similar to properties of sebum/ sebaceous oil.

The first major benefit of jojoba oil is that it acts as a moisturizer and hair conditioner. The sebaceous glands found on the scalp normally produce skin oil known as sebum that has the same structure like jojoba oil. The hair and scalp requires sebum to keep them moisturized and thus helps in maintaining healthy and beautiful hair while also reducing loss of hair. Jojoba oil comes with the same qualities offered by sebum oil and using jojoba oil regularly helps in improving the resistance of the hair to a range of detrimental factors like split ends, dryness and tangles.

It is also worth noting that you can also apply jojoba oil on the hair as a pure product and offers incredible benefits. Alternatively, you can but the oil as a component in other beauty products. It is advisable that you opt for the mixture as it also contains other extracts like rosemary oil, lavender and comfrey. Not only does your hair benefit from jojoba oil alone but will also benefit greatly from effects of the other extracts that offer more nourishment while healing the hair. For additional beauty and to deal with the problem of female pattern hair loss, the oil also offers numerous benefits of miniaturization, improved capillary circulation of the scalp and cleansing which improve follicle growth.

Jojoba oil also offers incredible benefits when applied on coarse and dry hair. In fact, jojoba oil not only works great in treating dry and coarse hair, but you can also use it repeatedly without any undesirable side effects on the hair. What makes the oil great is that it doesn't contain any chemicals in its content. In addition, applying jojoba oil can also be done easily and shampooing out is also easy. In fact, you don't have to worry about shampooing your head when trying to remove oil spots sticking on it as jojoba oil produces awesome effects when used on its own.

Using jojoba oil also gives you the benefit of healing and extra protection on your hair. Compounded with its awesome conditioning effects that naturally make your hair silky and soft, it would be a wise decision to choose hair loss products containing the oil. Scientific proof showing the healing properties of jojoba oil exists and can transform your hair positively than other ordinary oils. To top up on this, you can use jojoba oil on any kind of hair and still enjoy great results. There are many hair loss treatments on the marketing containing jojoba oil as a key ingredient in different concentrations to cater for your hair loss and miniaturization needs.

12.8 Emu Oil

Emu oil is natural oil that is derived from Australian Emu bird. Previous researchers and testimonials about emu oil show that it not only stops loss of hair in just 30 days but also promotes hair re-growth. Believe it or not, this sterilized oil produced from the fat of the Australian bird can be a sound solution to hair loss problems. You will be amazed by the incredible great results of this oil. The emu bird is found in Australia only and it is a large and flightless bird. Emu meat is marketed all over the world as a great low fat alternative for beet and the oil is one of the by-products during production of the meat. The oil goes through a refining process where all organic substances and traces of oil are removed.

A London journal explained that in 1860s, early settles in Australia used emu oil extensively for reducing pain, relieving muscular disorders and healing wounds. Even earlier than this, aboriginal Australians were reported to be using the emu oil for such and many other purposes. Today, one of the most popular hair loss treatments is emu oil thanks to its incredible healing properties and its remarkable potential of stimulating re-growth of lost hair in a matter of weeks. Emu oil can be used by both women and men alike. It is used as an alternative to drug treatments like Finasteride and Rogaine used for combating loss of hair.

The fact that makes emu oil a better alternative than other drug treatments is that while these treatments take years to deal with hair loss issues, emu oil offers better results in just a few weeks. In addition, emu oil also has the ability to prevent recurrence of loss of hair and eliminates the worries of having to use medical treatments forever. Additionally, another reason why you should consider using emu oil over these treatments is the issue of cost. Nowadays, drugs are pricey but emu oil is one of the cheapest yet very effective treatments for loss of hair.

With emu oil for hair loss, you also don't have to worry about undesirable side effects like groin pain, decreased sex drive and weight gain associated with other treatments. Ultimately, Finasteride and Minoxidil are not completely effective as they do not address the actual factors behind loss of hair. The effectiveness of emu oil lies on its ability to wake up most of the sleeping hair follicles that retards hair growth.

By using emu oil, the hair follicles become much more robust and there is a remarkable increase in skin thickness. This shows that the oil is able to stimulate the growth of both hair and the skin. As the oil awakes sleeping follicles, the hair is able to start growing all over again. Emu oil contains essential fatty acids in abundance including oleic acid that increases the ability of the oil penetrate the skin deeply. For best results, emu oil should be applied regularly on the scalp and incredible hair growth results will be seen within few weeks.

12.9 Licorice Herbal Remedy

The medicinal power and healing ability of licorice has been used since historical times in enhancing the health of hair/ scalp. In fact, ancient Egyptians came to discover about licorice and its incredible hair treatment benefits in 3rd century BC. Licorice basically contains a key compound which prevents testosterone hormone from being converted to DHT. This hormone is known to kill hair follicles and leads to development of male pattern baldness. As such, licorice shampoos are mainly used for bald prevention and offer a perfect solution for dealing with hair loss.

While licorice has a positive effect on growth of your hair, you should keep in mind the fact that male pattern baldness has no cure. However, using this herbal remedy on a daily basis promotes the health of your scalp and hair. Licorice is known to harbor regenerative properties and other essential compounds that boost hair growth. This herbal remedy helps to combat itchy, dry and irritated scalp and also reduces dandruffs on the scalp while promoting healthy hair growth and stopping hair loss. For people suffering from hair loss problems, licorice is a medication sent from heaven. In addition, its incredible healing properties also benefit people suffering from chemical or heat damage on the scalp and even scalp psoriasis. When applied gently on the scalp, licorice produces a minty tingle which heals, encourages and stimulates hair growth.

Conventionally, people treat hair loss using hair loss lotions, drugs, creams, surgeries and light therapy. However, licorice offers a much better alternative which guaranteeing superb results. Some of the other popular herbal remedies used alongside licorice include saw palmetto, stinging nettle, rosemary, grape seed, horsetail and green tea extracts which promotes scalp health and overall hair growth. Licorice root for hair loss is native to Australia, Eurasia, South and North America. This herb is estimated to be available in about 20 species and normally grows as a small shrub with pinnate leaves. The root of the herb/ shrub is used for treating loss of hair.

Traditional Chinese medicine used the roots of licorice for treating a range of different hair problems. When extracts of licorice root are taken in rather small amounts, they served as an effective tonic to adrenal glands. In addition, licorice is also used in form of a dietary supplement by people suffering from stomach ulcers, sore throat and bronchitis. The roots of licorice are rich in fats, protein, essential oils, amines, flavonoids, phytoestrogens, potassium, phosphorous, choline and B complex vitamins. These compounds and elements are very effective in promoting the health of scalp and entire hair.

Specifically, licorice enhances the effects of estrogen in the body which creates all this difference. Root extracts of this herb are very useful in treating dandruffs and improving growth of hair. You can also find licorice being sold in stores as tablets and capsules. However, taking licorice in large dosage should be avoided as this can lead to increased blood pressure, reduced levels of potassium, water retention and can also cause heart ailments.

12.10 Sage

Hair care specialists hail treatments such as sage for healthy hair growth as top options for alternative hair care and treatment. The sage leaf is known to contain a myriad of numerous beauty and healthy benefits. Oil contained in sage leaf gets extracted and is used in production of skin care products. In addition, the popular sage spice is extracted from dry sage leaves and is sprinkled on top of food as a way of enhancing flavor. Using sage spice or oil regularly helps to improve the renewal process of the skin and results in development of healthier hair and skin.

To start with sage oil improves scalp health. Massaging the oil on scalp stimulates renewal of dead cells and boosts circulation of blood. This herb is incredibly rich in both vitamin A and calcium which are essential for cell regeneration. Sage oil prevents appearance of the unsightly wrinkles and varicose veins which might appear prominently on the head. Sage extracts helps in reducing cellulite as well. Through promotion of increased supply of blood, sage assists in elimination of toxins the body stores which in turn prevents and reduces cellulite appearance. By massaging the scalp several times in a week, this helps in unlocking toxins trapped in the body and fat cells which can result in unsightly condition. By massaging your head with butter that contains sage oil, its cellulite reducing properties are directly absorbed in affected areas.

Most importantly, sage oil promotes growth of healthy hair. To achieve a healthy hair growth, you must use products of high quality and groom your hair properly. Products containing sage helps in improving the condition of brittle or weak hair and thankfully, sage assists in controlling secretion of oil in the body and minimizes the presence of oily hair. You can massage sage oil on the scalp directly, an activity that helps in increasing the flow of blood to hair follicles. This also encourages growth of healthy hair and also reduces loss of hair at the same time. In addition, sage is well known to be an effective natural reducer of gray hair.

The essential sage oil also has other valuable health benefits besides promoting growth of healthy hair which include aiding digestive disorders, acne, female complaints, boils, excess sebum and skin wrinkles. Sage oil is bactericidal, antispasmodic, antiseptic, carminative, euphoric, deodorant, nervine tonic and sedative properties. Going by this, it is pretty clear that sage offers valuable benefits in the world of natural medicine. To add on this, it is also evident that for people who are worried of getting old and appearance of gray hair, use of sage can bring an end to such worries.

Proper grooming and a healthy lifestyle enable the hair and skin to stay prepared to cope with external stressors that they face on a daily basis from the surrounding environment. Thankfully, sage oil can help you in having a blemish free and smooth screen while guaranteeing that your hair stays at its best condition possible.

12.11 Sunflower Oil

Otherwise known as Helianthus annulus, sunflower is a plant that is used to produce sunflower oil. This oil is derived from seeds of the beautiful, bright yellow sunflower. Sunflower oil comes packed with useful minerals and vitamins. In addition, the oil also contains unsaturated omega 6 fatty acids and linolenic acid. Due to this composition, sunflower oil offers incredible health benefits. Most importantly, the oil helps in treating various skin conditions, lowering cholesterol and high blood pressure, preventing migraines, heads and hear diseases as well as inflammation and asthma. Besides, sunflower oil is used in making of cosmetics, cooking oil and hair care products.

This oil also contains a myriad of essential nutrients like vitamins A, B6, B5 and B1 and vitamin E. The same sunflower oil is a host of numerous minerals that includes iron and folate, calcium and potassium. This oil which appears in a light yellow color can be applied on the hair directly where it acts as a very effective hair conditioner. Commercial hair products like hair pomade, hair conditioners and shampoos also contains sunflower as a key ingredient. When used in hair care, sunflower oil adds shine and luster while also protecting your hair against the harmful ultra violet sun rays. In addition, the oil also gives your hair a soft and smooth feeling besides giving it a beautiful, luxuriant appearance.

Sunflower oil is known to act as a moisturizer or an emollient and plays a key role in helping the skin to stay moist and supple. By keeping the scalp and hair moisturized, it prevents your skin from becoming dry flaky. Using sunflower oil on scalp and hair or using hair care products containing the oil prevents loss of moisture from the hair and ensures that the scalp doesn't become dry flaky. In the long run, your hair gets a healthy appearance and looks shiny as well. Apart from the moisturizing effects of sunflower oil, it is also known to have high contents of fatty acids and vitamins that condition and nourishes the scalp and hair. Also, thanks to the presence of ultraviolet protection filter, sunflower also helps the hair to retain its color and ensures that it stays at its best.

In addition, using sunflower oil has been found to be very beneficial in treating hair thinning. Scientists also say that sunflower oil contains gamma linolenic acid or GLA in high levels. Other clinical studies have also noted that the oil has high levels of omega 6 fatty acids that assist in preventing loss of hair and also stimulating growth of thicker and healthier hair. Besides consuming sunflower oil supplements, you should also apply the oil on your scalp which conditions and nourishes hair follicles. The same oil also makes your hair follicles remain strong and stay healthy while also producing thicker, fuller and shiner hair strands. Sunflower has been tested and found effective in stopping activities of DHT that can trigger loss of hair and hair thinning.

12.12 Rosemary

Even though rosemary is well known as a spice in seasoning food like sausage, poultry, stews and soups, it is no longer a secret that rosemary is a highly effective treatment for hair loss. To be more precise, rosemary slows down the progression of premature loss of hair by stimulating hair follicles and thus promotes better hair health. Besides, hair experts also say that this herbal remedy is also very valuable in relieving dandruffs and itchy, dry scalp.

Even for those with a perfectly normal hair, using rosemary will leave it shiny and soft. There are many commercial hair products sold in online stores that contain rosemary and besides, you can also prepare a home treatment of rosemary at the comfort of your home using the leaves of this herb.

Naturalists agree that rosemary is one of the most powerful herbs and offers a multitude of significant health benefits. Rosemary oil and rosemary tea are extensively used in normal hair care routines and for great reasons. Existing organic facts confirm that rosemary oil stimulate the hair follicles and makes the hair to grow strong and long. In addition, rosemary fights premature loss of hair and prevents hair from falling when shampooing, brushing or just going about your daily business.

More precisely, this herbal remedy has been found to be more beneficial for women suffering from hormonal related hair loss or PCOS, people who are worried about balding and people suffering from alopecia areata. For people who are also worried about fighting hair graying issues, rosemary is also able to deal with that effectively. The herbal remedy also promotes hair pigmentation and prevents hair from graying prematurely and in some cases; researchers have found that rosemary can reverse grey hair. By using the oil regularly, you will be fascinated to see your grey hairs slowly disappear from your head.

A flaky, dry scalp is mostly a result of dandruffs and thankfully, rosemary acts as a good natural remedy for this as well. The oil has very strong disinfecting and detoxifying attributes and when these are combined with the invigorating attributes of rosemary, you are assured of having a flake free and healthy hair and scalp with regular usage.

According to scientists and researchers, rosemary is able to accomplish all these through its ability to boost circulation of blood in the scalp. When more blood flows into the scalp, the hair receives the much needed nutrients and oxygen to grow. This promotes renewed hair cellular health and your hair becomes fuller, shiny and much healthier.

Using rosemary oil is pretty easy and it is best done by directly applying it on the scalp. For the best results, you can even mix rosemary oil with other health herbal remedies like fenugreek, bhringraj, sage, aloe Vera and horsetail. Besides this, you can as well use rosemary in form of tea and rinse your hair with it. This way, you will be amazed by how rosemary can make a tremendous improvement on the health of your hair and scalp.

12.13 Ginko Biloba

Hair loss can be triggered by numerous factors including scalp disease, unhealthy diet, poor scalp circulation, pollution, genetics, poor quality shampoos and hormonal imbalances among other factors. Our hair becomes more vulnerable to degradation and breakage the more it is exposed to pollutants and air particles. In such circumstances, Ginko biloba functions as the best solution for hair loss. This herbal remedy is widely acclaimed to have originated from China and it is a critical aspect of the traditional Chinese medicine. For the past two centuries, the western world has come to accept the extracts of Ginko biloba tree as highly valuable in treatment of a wide range of health problems especially in promoting healthy hair growth.

Ginko biloba is believed to contain special ingredients which when administered in the body they provide the blood with fresh impetus which enhances proper promotion. As such, Ginko biloba promotes growth of healthy hair by boosting circulation and transportation of essential nutrients to the scalp and hair for growth. Normally, one of the factors that lead to loss of hair is poor scalp circulation. However, some herbal remedies like Ginko biloba and Cayenne pepper have proved to be very effective in reversing this situation.

Ginko biloba helps in strengthening the heart which makes it strong enough to pump blood to the furthest corners in the human blood. This way, this herb increases circulation of blood to and from different parts of the human body including the head region which houses the brain, scalp and hair follicles. With improved circulation thanks to Ginko biloba, diseases like thrombosis, Reynaud's phenomenon and hair loss are rectified. In addition, improved circulation of blood in the body promotes overall health wellness and ensures that your body is free from common problems and diseases.

Ginko biloba speeds up the flow of blood to important body peripherals that might not receive sufficient blood circulation under ordinary circumstances. As such, capillaries that supply the scalp with blood receive blood in abundance. Since this blood contains oxygen, increased blood supply means that the hair will automatically receive more oxygen which is essential for growth. Besides nutrients, oxygen also carries along essential vitamins like A and E that give the hair a new lease of life.

Once the human scalp receives these supplies in abundance, they promote repair of damaged hair and re-growth of lost hair. As such, Ginko biloba is what you need for your hair to appear bouncy, silky and healthy.

12.14 Cider Vinegar

Thanks to its effectiveness, cider vinegar is a natural remedy that helps in eliminating the embarrassment that comes with having a big bald spot on your forehead. Nowadays, there are so many natural treatments which guarantee to reduce loss of hair and make your hair grow healthier. Nevertheless, vinegar is with no doubt one of the most valuable home remedy which assists in making your hair look fuller and healthier once again.

For most women and men alike, hair is their pride and it is always a quite painful experience to see the hair start to fall slowly by slowly. However, cider vinegar helps avoid this first by guaranteeing you a healthy scalp which is one of the most important things when thinking about preventing hair loss and hair thinning. Actually, the nature of your scalp determines whether taking cider vinegar is going to be a successful or not. In fact, most of the hair treatments and hair growth products being sold on the market today aim at making sure that the pores stay open so that they can pave a way for development and growth of new hair. Cider vinegar is one of the most beneficial natural remedies that aids in keeping the scalp cleared in order to promote hair growth while ensuring that your hair stays at its healthiest state possible.

In addition, cider vinegar stimulates growth of hair follicles. By using the herbal remedy regularly, you have a high chance of making your hair stronger and healthier by countering the side effects of insufficient blood circulation in the body. Vinegar improved better blood circulation from your body to the hair follicles. The process of blood circulation in the body is critical and of significant importance as it ensures that the scalp and hair follicles obtain essential nutrients and oxygen needed for growth. Normally, people with an efficient circulation of blood tend to have healthy and strong hair as presence of essential nutrients makes the roots of hair follicles stronger.

Another pretty thing about cider vinegar is that it eliminates build up that inhibits hair growth. Basically, the hair has its natural PH level which can at times drop from 5 to 4. When you mix some cider vinegar with water and apply it gently on your scalp, you are able to keep your scalp's PH level in control. In addition, washing the hair in such a mixture also helps in eliminating build up that could be clogging in your hair and preventing its growth. Most of the hair treatment and supplements sold today are alkaline in nature and this can have some detrimental effects on your hair. Thankfully, cider vinegar helps to neutralize alkaline and highly acidic shampoos that can make your hair dry, brittle and break off more easily.

13. Surgical Treatments

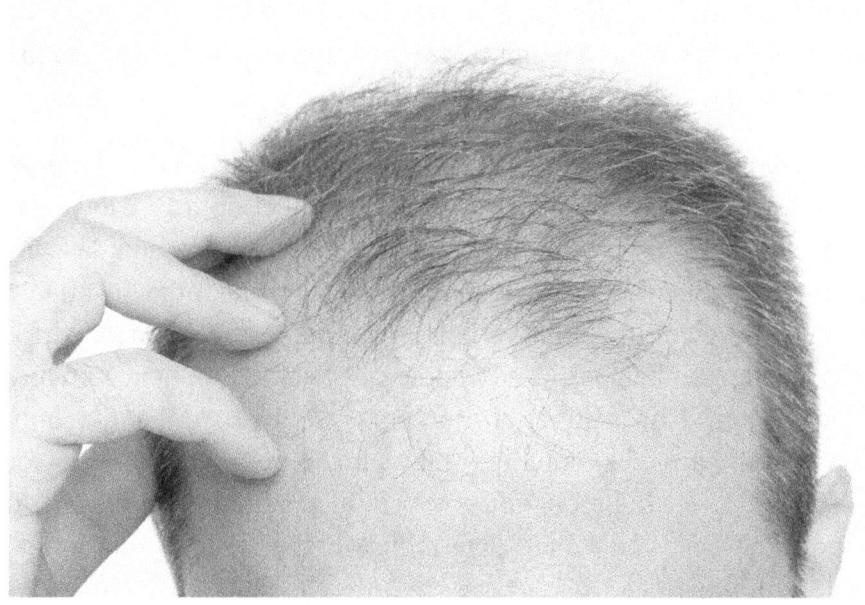

Surgical hair loss treatment offers a permanent solution to people suffering from hair loss and hair thinning problems. If you can afford this treatment, you have nothing to worry about hair loss as the condition can be fixed once and for all through surgery. Fortunately, surgical hair restoration has multiple payment and financing options which makes the procedure more affordable. Third party credit agencies provide candidates of hair transplantation with numerous financing options to meet the cost of the procedure.

Surgical treatment for hair loss involves the removal of individual follicles from the donor site- the sides or back of head- where the hair has more resistance to balding and thinning. The hair removed is then transplanted to other areas of your head experiencing baldness and thinning where their growth continues naturally. In most cases, hair loss among men and women is largely attributed to DHT hormone and during hair transplantation; the hair follicles that are resistant to DHT are removed from scalp and then artfully placed on areas experiencing thinning. The front and top of the head are the areas that mostly require transplantation.

Hair transplantation as a form of hair loss and hair thinning transplantation has incredible options than other options. However, to go through this procedure, you must be the right candidate for transplant otherwise you might have to consider other available options. Surgical treatment of hair loss is highly recommended for men who are in their early and middle stages of loss of hair. Actually, even though hair restoration surgery is known to be the only permanent hair loss solution, this procedure is not meant for everyone. As such, before you embrace this procedure as the end to your hair woes, you should determine whether it is an appropriate option for you.

Ideally, men suffering from male pattern baldness or genetic hair loss are the best candidates to go for a hair transplant surgery. Men with male pattern baldness are normally characterized by a receding hair line or loss of hair at the crown and sometimes both. Hair transplantation cost is a critical factor to factor in for any person thinking of hair replacement options. As you evaluate a typical hair transplant surgery, you should know how much the procedure is going to cost you. Generally, the cost of hair transplantation is based on 'per graft'. As such, you get to pay based on your personal hair replacement needs.

Due to how hair transplantation cost is determined, it is hard to get an estimation over the phone or online. Instead, you should consider scheduling a no obligation appointment with a hair specialist to get your condition assessed. Normally, the doctor will price the procedure based on the amount of hair that you have lost so far, the amount of the donor hair available and the characteristic of donor hair based on texture, curl and color. Finally, your desired results will also determine the overall cost of the procedure.

Even though your individual requirements will determine the overall cost, there is of course the average cost of the procedure that you should expect to pay. There are some hair loss patients who opt to go for different procedures so that they can achieve their own personal goals. However, you should know that the long run 'cost per graft' decreases as you have more hairs being transplanted. Generally, the cost of hair restoration surgery is $5-10/graft depending on many factors such as the number of hair grafts being done and how good the surgeon is.

As a hair transplantation candidate, it is of paramount importance that you choose the right hair restoration surgeon. The end results will be determined by the skills, talent and experience of the surgeon. As such, you need to research widely and pick your doctor wisely by considering a wide range of factors like reviews, patient testimonials and cost of the procedure.

13.1 Hair Transplant Surgery Procedure

Here is a well detailed, step by step procedure of what you should expect when you go for a hair transplant surgery. The timeline of the procedure spans from before, during and after the hair transplantation surgery. First, before your procedure, you should have a good rest at night. This means that you limit your alcohol and smoking and ensure that you take a healthy breakfast. For several days before the hair transplant material day, you will be asked not to use aspirin. You should discuss with your physician for more details depending on your specific condition.

On the day of procedure, arrive at the clinic as per your scheduled time. Hair transplant surgery is basically an outpatient procedure with lasts between 3 and 8 hours. However, in rare situations, the entire procedure can take much longer even though this will depend on the follicular units to be transplanted. You should be relaxed during the procedure. The first step is donor area preparation. The doctor will take a donor strip from the side or back of your head where your hair is resistant to being lost genetically. The hair near the donor strip will be secured or taped as the donor area gets trimmed. During this procedure, a local anesthetic will be used to numb the area.

The next step is harvesting of hair and this is done by surgically removing the skin on donor area. After healing, there will be a fine scar or cosmetic line left and existing hair on the head will cover it. In fact, even immediately after the donor area is sutured, you can hardly see the affected area. The third step is separation where a team of medical assistances will work with stereo microscopes to divide the donor hair strip hair and group it into natural follicles. Naturally, the hair tends to grow in groupings comprising of between one and four hairs.

Next, the hair specialist will create recipient sites and this step is more artistic rather than medication. During the procedure, the doctor makes incisions on the hair follicles and this follows exact angle and direction of your normal hair growth. When creating these recipient sites, the medical personnel must be well experienced.

The final step of the procedure is placing. The follicular units prepared are placed carefully into recipients sites. At the front area, the medical team will usually place the 1 and 2 hair follicular groupings while other follicular units that include three to four hairs will be placed at the top of head in order to provide more density. After this procedure is over, the medical team should review the whole procedure the day after procedure where they will wash your hair. They will also give you a medical guide and kit on how you will take care of your transplanted hair especially for the first ten days which are more crucial. Once you have healed completely, no scarring will be visible and new hair will start growing naturally.

When it comes to the number of sessions needed for hair transplant surgery, hair transplantation sessions can be as many as necessary and depending on the needed hair follicles. For instance, if a patient requires 15000 hair strands, these can't be done in one session especially if you need qualified results. It is advisable that you get between 3000 and 4000 per session which averages between 3 and 4 hours. Sessions can be repeated after a week and all the hair strands will be transplanted completely may be within a month's time.

13.2 Recovery Process

How first you recover after hair replacement surgery depends on complexity and extent of the procedure. Once the hair transplantation process is completed there are other critical post operative steps which you should follow in order to enhance a speedy recovery process and also minimize the risk of damaging your newly implanted hair follicles. The physician will prescribe to you pain medications that will help in controlling any aching, throbbing or excessive tightness. It is common for patients to be given a post-operative pack containing medicine such as mild pain relievers and antibiotics that they need as they recover. Some also give the patient some mild sedatives to help them sleep comfortably for the first few days as the scalp is normally tender and there is a bit of discomfort. The surgeon will also advise you to remove the bandages after a day and after two days; you can wash the hair gently. Between 7 and 10 days, you will need to have the stitches remove.

During the recovery procedure, there is a possibility of experiencing drainage, bruising and swelling which you need to discuss with the surgeon. Strenuous activities can hamper the recovery procedure by increasing the flow of blood to the scalp and causing the incisions or transplants to bleed. As such, you should avoid vigorous exercises during your recovery period especially in the first three weeks. Some surgeons will also advise you not to engage in sexual activities after surgery during the first 10 days. The doctor will also advise you to visit his clinic for check-ups to ensure that the incisions are recovering properly.

For the first two weeks after surgery, you should avoid exposing your head to direct sunlight. To reduce the chances of swelling, it is essential that you use about two pillows when sleeping and if possible, use a recliner chair for sleeping. Formation of scabs during healing and recovery period is natural and you should leave them on their own. For speedy and successful recovery, there are certain things that you need to avoid. For instance scratching the hair grafts where the transplantation was done might end up compromising the results. However, you should give the area a light massage to enhance the recovery.

To minimize itchiness, it is advisable that you apply 1 percent hydrocortisone cream twice in a day. If you do smoke, you are advised highly to stop the habit especially for the first week of recovery. Smoking leads to constriction of blood vessels which slows supply of blood to implanted grafts. Smoking also decreases amount of oxygen available in the scalp which inhibits quick healing. After the first 10 days, the pain should be gone even though you might still be experiencing some numbness which should disappear by the end of second week.

During the recovery period, you will to shampoo and cleanse the shampoo to remove crusts and minimize infection risk. It is important to avoid soaking your hair in a lot of water during the cleansing as this can lead to swelling. To give your results a more natural look, you might need to go for a touch up surgical procedure after healing of the incisions. Sometimes, the follow up procedure involve blending where the hairline is filled using slit grafts, micro-grafts or mini- grafts. Your doctor should assess you and advise on whether you need any touch up procedure after recovery or not.

13.3 Caring for Your Hair After Surgery

After undergoing hair transplant surgery procedure, there are a few things you should do for the best results to be achieved. Taking good care of your transplanted hair is important as this promotes fast healing and helps you achieve your desired expectations. First, you will need to take the medication as recommended by your doctor. You will be given a prescription of several medicines which will promote healing of the transplants. Normally, the medicines given will be anti-inflammatory and anti-biotic drugs. Antibiotics prevents infection while anti-inflammatory pills minimizes pain that could result from the incisions.

Dressing the wound should be done strictly as advised by the doctor. Most importantly, you should keep your wound sterile and a cotton or gaze soaked in an antiseptic solution such as alcohol will be of great use. Applying this formula should be done between 2 and 3 times in a day in order to remove the sutures fully. Dressing the wound promotes fast healing. Also sleep in a manner that the pillow doesn't press the wound otherwise you might move the wound and lead to scattering of blood on the pillow. If you start bleeding, make sure that you apply an antiseptic solution with cotton and the bleeding gets to stop.

The food and drink you eat also play a major role in your after care treatment. Actually, you are not restrained to eat specific foods and you are at liberty of choosing what you want to eat. However, you should keep off alcohol as alcohol does not react favorably with most medications. Alcohol is also a depressant which can seriously interfere with your recovery process. Actually, caring for your hair after surgery is not restrictive but it is essential that you use common sense to avoid complications.

After the surgery, do not comb the hair and you should discontinue using your normal products unless the doctor advises you otherwise. Shampoos and commercial hair products can infect and irritate the incisions. In addition, scratching the head should be avoided. To minimize the itching effect, most doctors recommend the use of topical ointments approved for that purpose. Itching is likely to happen as holes form scabs which fight bacteria intruding the wounds. As such, experiencing itching means that you are on the right track of healing.

Sun bathing is also highly discouraged after hair transplantation as well as going to sauna and exposing yourself to any kind of heat. Exposing your head to a hot environment simply increases the inflammation; do not forget that warmer environment makes bacteria to multiply much faster. You should also avoid performing exercises until you are sure that the wounds have healed. If you are a weight lifter, you should refrain from such activities especially in the first month. If you must engage in strenuous exercises, do so gradually. This is because such activities increases pressure on transplanted area and can lead to bursting of blood vessels which will obviously slow down the healing process.

About the Author

Jonathan Affleck is a hair health expert and writer. He is the author of two books: Hair Loss Solutions: Causes, Prevention and Treatments and The Consumer's Guide to Hair Transplant. He is dedicated his career to helping people understand and treat hair loss problems.